the

LITTLE BOOK

of

Marilyn

INSPIRATION FROM THE

GODDESS *of* GLAM

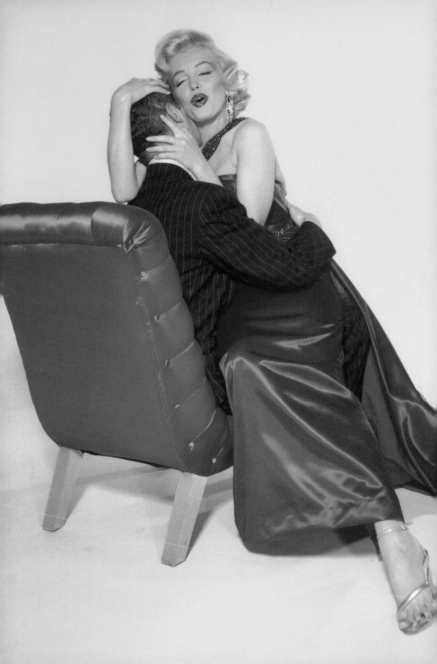

the
LITTLE BOOK
of
Marilyn
INSPIRATION FROM THE
GODDESS *of* GLAM

by MICHELLE MORGAN

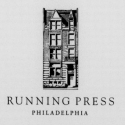

RUNNING PRESS
PHILADELPHIA

Running Press
Hachette Book Group
1290 Avenue of the Americas, New York, NY 10104
www.runningpress.com
@Running_Press

Printed in China

First Edition: July 2019

Published by Running Press, an imprint of Perseus Books, LLC, a subsidiary of Hachette Book Group, Inc. The Running Press name and logo is a trademark of the Hachette Book Group.

The Hachette Speakers Bureau provides a wide range of authors for speaking events. To find out more, go to www.hachettespeakersbureau.com or call (866) 376-6591.

The publisher is not responsible for websites (or their content) that are not owned by the publisher.

Print book cover and interior design by Susan Van Horn.

Library of Congress Control Number: 2018964554

ISBNs: 978-0-7624-6654-2 (flexibound), 978-0-7624-6653-5 (ebook)

1010

10 9 8 7 6 5 4 3 2 1

For Aunty Dawn—
I couldn't have written this
book without you.
And for Maureen Brown—
my dear friend and fellow
Marilyn fan.

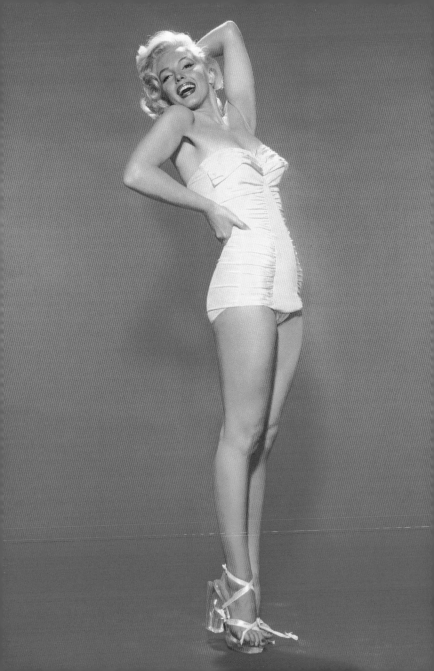

contents

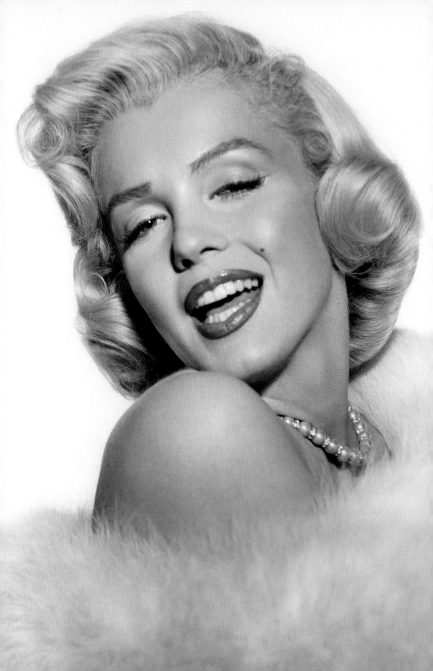

introduction

I first truly discovered Marilyn Monroe on a postcard stand in Devon, England, during a seaside holiday in 1985. I had been aware of her before, of course, and she had been more visible on my radar since Madonna performed as her in the video for "Material Girl." However, the postcard of Marilyn in a gold-lamé dress, blowing a kiss at the camera, triggered something inside me. At a time when I felt like the most unglamorous person in the world, Marilyn's beauty, style, and sophistication spoke to my teenage heart. The next day I bought a biography of her to read on the beach. I was excited to know more about this beautiful woman, but I had absolutely no idea just how important she would become to me.

I was fifteen years old, unconfident and unsure of what I wanted to do with my life. It was also the era of playground politics for me—that depressing time when friendships are broken on an almost daily basis and when one person falls out with you, the rest of the group seems to follow. I started

OPPOSITE: In the 1980s, this photograph was a staple for any teenage girl's bedroom.

1

summer vacation feeling fairly **unhappy, but** after discovering Marilyn and applying **some of her attitude** to my own life, I returned to school in **September quite** transformed. A glimpse at my 1985 journal confirms **that** I was taken aback by how much my outlook had **changed,** just by learning about Marilyn and adopting a few elements of her style.

In the thirty-three years that have passed since then, I've discovered that many people—men as well as women—have been greatly inspired by Marilyn. Some enjoy dressing as her, while others take comfort in watching her films or learning about her life and career. There are even collectors lucky enough to buy her personal belongings at auction. But whatever kind of devotee you are, we all have something in common: Marilyn has enriched our existence in ways we never thought possible.

A celebration of the fans as well as the star, *The Little Book of Marilyn* presents a mixture of inspiration, tutorials, and crafts, which will enable us all to put a bit more Marilyn into our lives.

Let's get started!

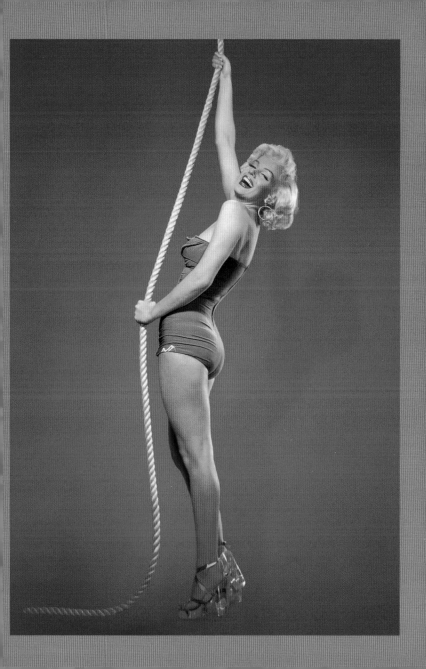

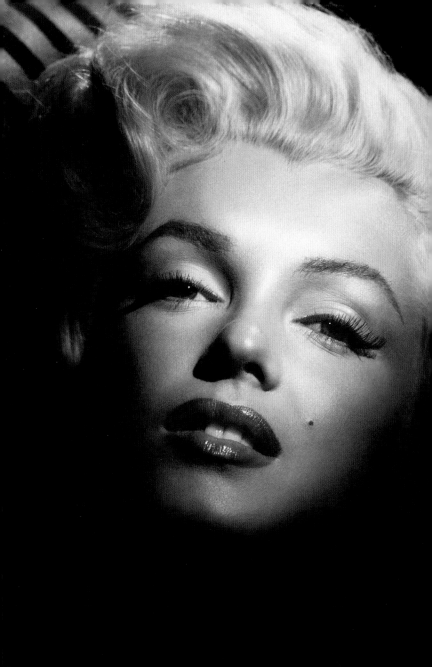

ONE

her story

ONE OF THE MANY SOURCES OF INSPIRATION FOR Marilyn's supporters is the knowledge that while in her early life she was often sad and despondent, she was able to rise up and become one of the most successful women in the world. Born Norma Jeane Mortenson (changed shortly after to Baker), she was the daughter of Gladys, a twice-divorced film cutter for Consolidated Industries. Her father was believed to be Charles Stanley Gifford, a boss at Consolidated, though for years Norma Jeane was unaware of his identity and spent most of her childhood believing her father was deceased.

Unable to cope with the demands of motherhood and a full-time job, Gladys enlisted the help of her mother's neighbors the Bolenders to care for Norma Jeane. The couple fostered other children, and for a time the situation worked out well. The child stayed with the family, while Gladys divided her time between working in Hollywood and traveling to see her daughter. Unfortunately, life had been hard for Gladys, and she suffered from a variety of problems, including mental illness. Even though she attempted the role of Norma Jeane's full-time guardian in the mid-1930s, her emotional state was fragile. After a breakdown, Gladys was admitted to a psychiatric hospital, and her

OPPOSITE: Norma Jeane with her mother in the late 1920s. PREVIOUS SPREAD: An unusual and beautiful studio close-up.

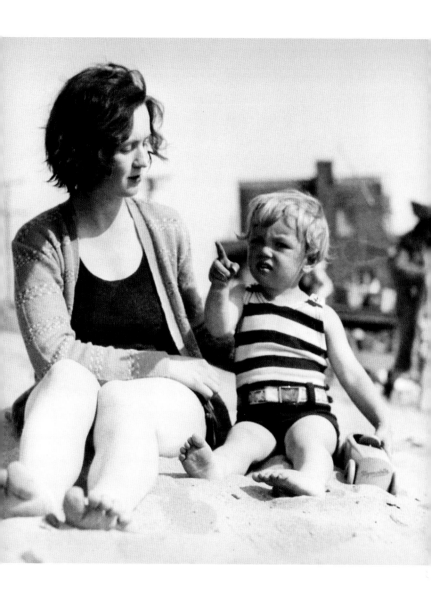

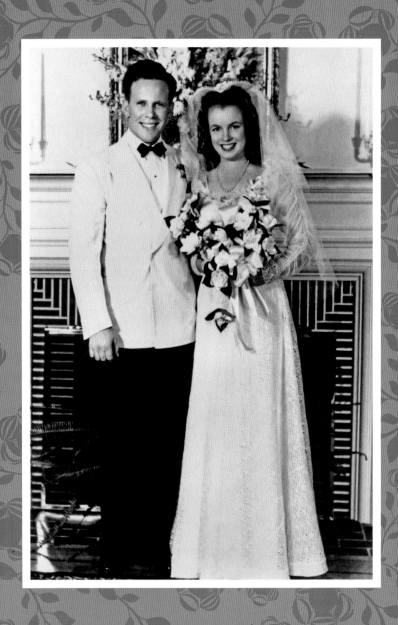

daughter spent the rest of her childhood being cared for by family friends, foster parents, and an orphanage.

When Norma Jeane was fifteen, her current foster parents, the Goddards, planned to move away from Los Angeles and did not have the means (or permission) to take her with them. Not wanting to see the girl sent back to an orphanage, Mrs. Goddard conspired with a neighbor to encourage her son, James Dougherty, to date and then marry Norma Jeane. The plan worked perfectly, and the couple wed shortly after her sixteenth birthday, in June 1942. The couple settled down to married life, until James enlisted to fight for his country in the Merchant Marines and Norma Jeane somewhat reluctantly moved in with his parents.

Marilyn would later say that she really only married Dougherty in order to escape the orphanage. Letters show that she did have some feelings for her husband, but the girl was young and wanted more in her life than marriage and children. The chance for independence came when Norma Jeane began working in an ammunitions factory. While there she had her picture taken by a photographer named David Conover, who had been sent to snap women working for the war effort. He immediately saw a photogenic talent in Norma Jeane and introduced her to some photographer

OPPOSITE: Norma Jeane married neighbor James Dougherty to escape going back into an orphanage.

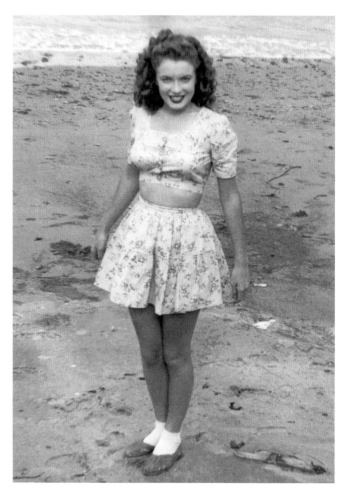

Norma Jeane poses on a beach at Catalina Island. Her modeling career was just around the corner. OPPOSITE: Starlet Marilyn Monroe attends a publicity event.

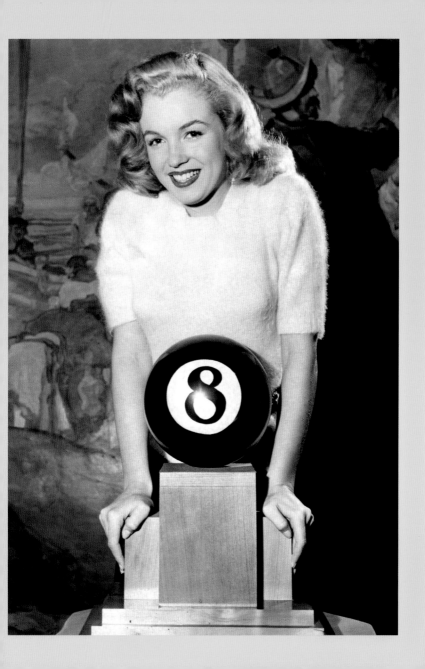

friends. Her talents were soon recognized, and it wasn't long before she was signed to the Blue Book Agency, headed by Emmeline Snively.

Norma Jeane's childhood had never been particularly positive, but her newfound career gave her boundless confidence, and she soon became a popular and very busy model. Her emergence as an independent, working woman ensured that her marriage to James Dougherty was over, especially when casting directors and producers took notice of her on magazine covers and began making enquiries about her availability as an actress.

In the latter half of 1946, Norma Jeane divorced her husband and was signed to Twentieth Century Fox. Casting director Ben Lyon deemed her name not interesting enough, and a new one was sought. Marilyn Miller was proposed, but the twenty-year-old did not care for the name and exclaimed that she didn't know how to spell Marilyn. A compromise was found when Norma Jeane suggested Monroe as a surname, since that had been her mother's maiden name. The studio agreed, and Marilyn Monroe was born.

Despite her enthusiasm, Marilyn's contract was not renewed after a year, and she was out of Twentieth Century Fox with only two tiny film appearances to her name.

OPPOSITE: The beach and swimwear were regular themes in publicity photos.

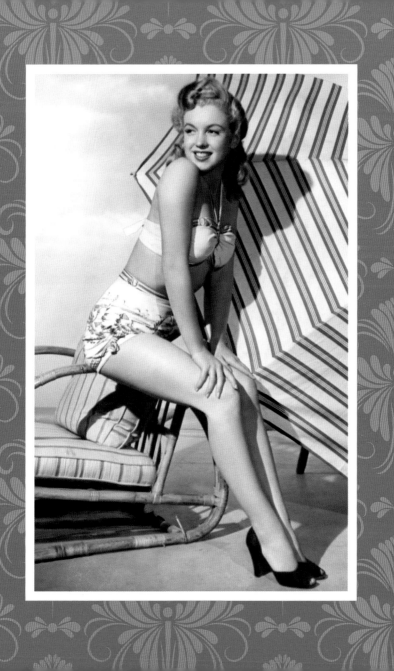

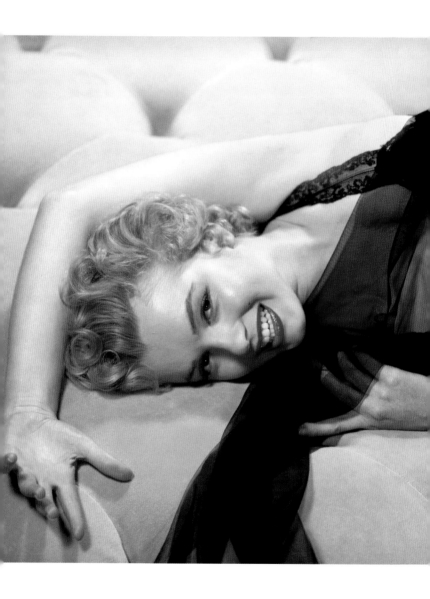

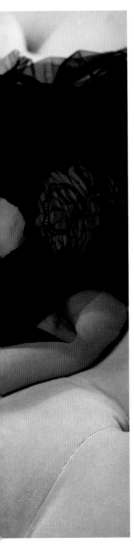

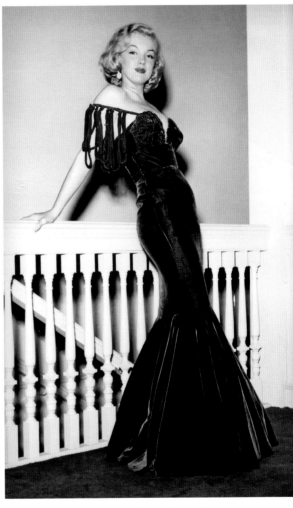

Low-cut gowns such as these often raised eyebrows in the early 1950s.

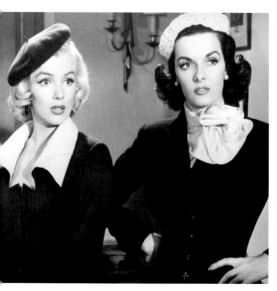 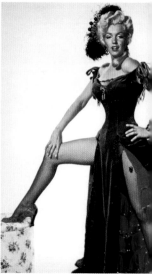

FROM LEFT: Marilyn and Jane Russell on the set of *Gentlemen Prefer Blondes*. • It was roles like this one in *River of No Return* that prompted Marilyn to start her own film company.

In order to pay the bills, she flitted between several other studios, went back to modeling, and posed for nude photographs by Tom Kelley. However, by the early 1950s she was back at Fox, and this time they signed the fledgling star to a long-term contract.

After the struggle of her early years, Marilyn's star rose quickly, thanks mainly to the fact that the public absolutely adored her, even in small roles. Letters poured into the

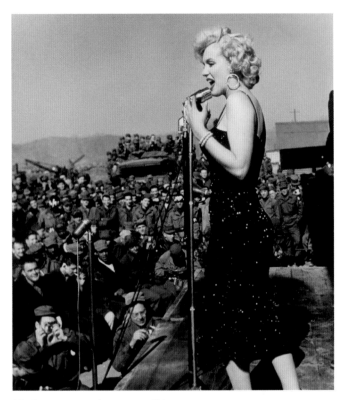

Marilyn entertains the troops in Korea in 1954.

studio on a daily basis, and gossip columnists were always keen to write about (and often champion) her career. Not even the discovery of Marilyn's nude calendar pictures in conservative 1950s America was enough to dim her sparkle, and the studio put her into as many films as it could.

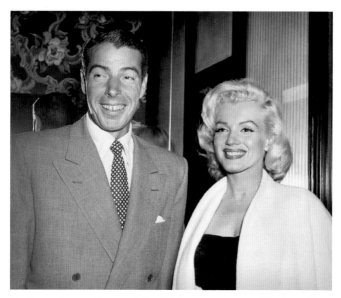

Marilyn and second husband, Joe DiMaggio. OPPOSITE: *The Seven Year Itch* skirt-blowing scene.

By 1954 Marilyn had appeared in blockbusters such as *Niagara*, *Gentlemen Prefer Blondes*, and *How to Marry a Millionaire*, but her magnificent success came at a price. Marilyn was an intelligent woman—an ambitious soul who read great literature and took night school classes—but the public's enjoyment of the succession of dumb blonde roles she played ensured the studio continued to see (and cast) her that way. Her marriage to baseball star Joe DiMaggio added another complication to her life and career ambitions, as

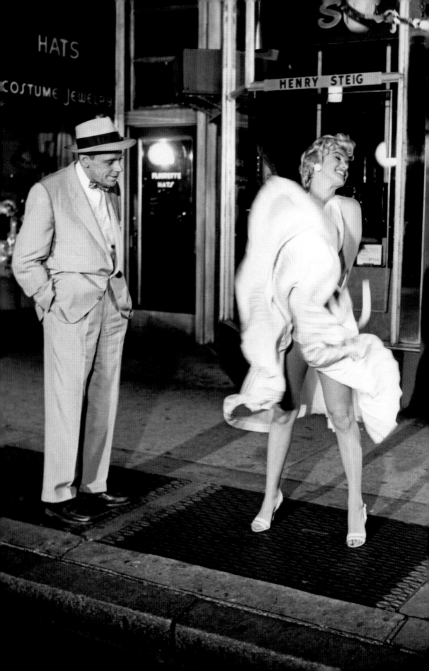

her new and somewhat jealous husband wrongly assumed that Marilyn would abandon her film work in order to become a full-time wife and mother.

The marriage between DiMaggio and Marilyn failed spectacularly after the filming of the immortal subway scene for *The Seven Year Itch*, which featured her skirt blowing above her knees amid a torrent of publicity. This pivotal event confirmed Joe's fears that Marilyn had no intention of kissing her career good-bye, and the couple parted shortly afterward, though they remained friends for the rest of her life. When *The Seven Year Itch* finished filming in late 1954, Marilyn rebelled against the studio's typecasting, walked out on her contract, flew to New York, and created her own film company with photographer Milton Greene. Her reasoning was that she wanted to act in dramatic parts as well as musicals, something Twentieth Century Fox was reluctant to let her do.

For a time Marilyn's ambitions were mocked by the studio and journalists alike. They wondered how the actress could possibly think of herself as an independent entity, when she was supposedly signed to Fox for the coming years. News that she was studying at the famed Actors Studio under the guidance of Lee and Paula Strasberg was met with even more derision.

20

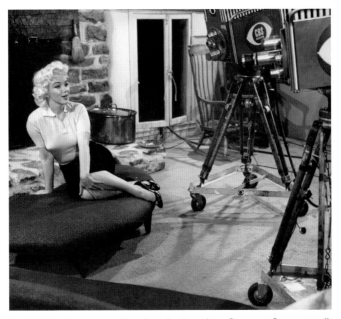

In 1955, Marilyn appeared on the television show *Person to Person* to talk about her new film company.

The idea that a so-called blonde bombshell could become a trailblazing businesswoman and actress was unthinkable to some, but Marilyn was full of surprises. She proved the naysayers wrong when, at the end of 1955, Twentieth Century Fox signed her to a revolutionary contract that enabled her to work with the studio and independently, too. She also had a say in what directors she would work for—a major achievement for an actress in the mid-1950s. This

21

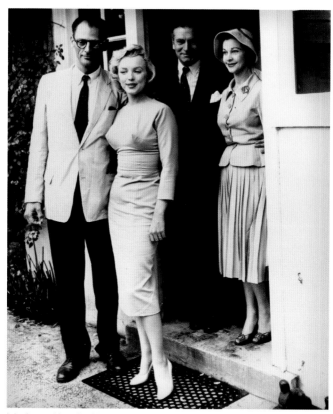

Marilyn and her third husband, Arthur Miller, shortly after arriving in London.

was just the beginning of a fascinating period of time, one that would see Marilyn star in the critically acclaimed movie *Bus Stop* and marry respected playwright Arthur Miller. Suddenly the tide began to turn: people realized that if Marilyn

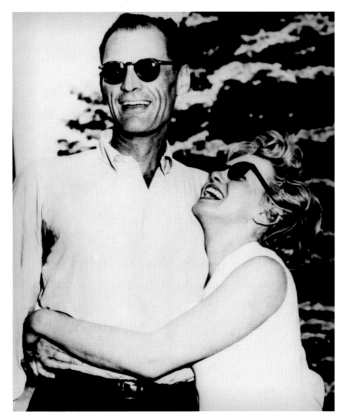

Looking casual, during her marriage to Arthur Miller.

Monroe could pull off such a magnificent performance in
Bus Stop, and a Pulitzer Prize–winning author could see her
as intellectually attractive, then maybe she wasn't a dumb
blonde after all.

She and Miller embarked on a trip to England to make *The Prince and the Showgirl* with Laurence Olivier. The two stars aggravated each other almost immediately, and by the time production finished, in November 1956, Marilyn was exceedingly happy to return to New York. There she took on the role of housewife to Miller and stepmother to his children, while trying desperately to create a family of her own. Sadly, her attempts at motherhood ended in miscarriage, first in the summer of 1957 and then toward the end of 1958, shortly after working on one of her most celebrated and popular films, *Some Like It Hot*.

In 1960, Marilyn had an affair with her married costar, Yves Montand, while on the set of *Let's Make Love*. The relationship only lasted the length of the shoot, and then she immediately went on to make the Miller-penned movie *The Misfits*. Shooting in the desert heat of Nevada was a nightmare for all concerned, particularly because Marilyn was often late on set and then became ill with extreme exhaustion and spent time in the hospital. Her marriage unraveled during filming, and by the time *The Misfits* wrapped, it was over.

The next year was a pivotal one for Marilyn, as she recovered from the emotional work on *The Misfits* and the

OPPOSITE, FROM TOP: Marilyn arrives in Nevada to make her last completed movie, *The Misfits*. • Marilyn signs autographs on the set of *The Misfits*.

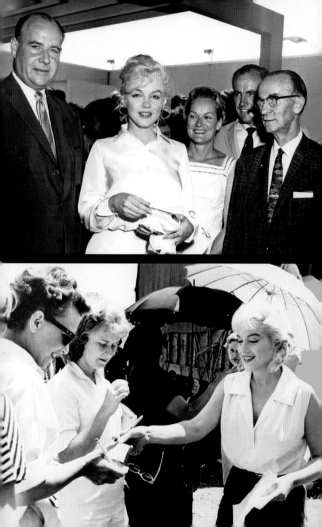

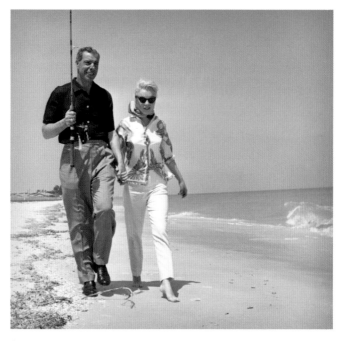

Second husband Joe DiMaggio proved to be a good friend in the last years of Marilyn's life.

strain of her separation from Arthur Miller. Early in 1961, the actress was admitted to the Payne Whitney Psychiatric Clinic in New York, though she always insisted that her doctor had tricked her into going there. Letters written from the hospital show that Marilyn was forced to sleep in a room with a glass door (so that doctors and nurses could observe her), and the bathroom was kept locked. When she was finally able to get in touch with ex-husband Joe DiMaggio, he stormed the hospital and insisted she be released into his care.

The remainder of 1961 was spent recovering from the stress of the past year. DiMaggio was often by her side, and rumors swirled that the two were about to remarry. Marilyn always denied such stories and insisted that Joe was purely a great friend. Putting the previous few years behind her, the actress decided to leave New York and return to Los Angeles. This was a pivotal time for Marilyn, not least because she decided to buy a house, rather than renting or living in hotels, as she had always done in Los Angeles. She bought a bungalow at 12305 Fifth Helena Drive, in the quiet neighborhood of Brentwood, and was optimistic for the future. The refurbishment of the home provided a distraction from her recent upsets, but an addiction to prescription medication and mental health problems such as depression and anxiety were frightening and recurring struggles for the star.

In addition, Twentieth Century Fox still seemed to resent Marilyn for the way she had left the studio in 1954, and tensions ran high on the set of her next movie, *Something's Got to Give*. Marilyn had been invited to sing at President John F. Kennedy's lavish birthday party at Madison Square Garden, but while she initially had permission to fly to New York, delays on set prompted Fox to pull the plug and

27

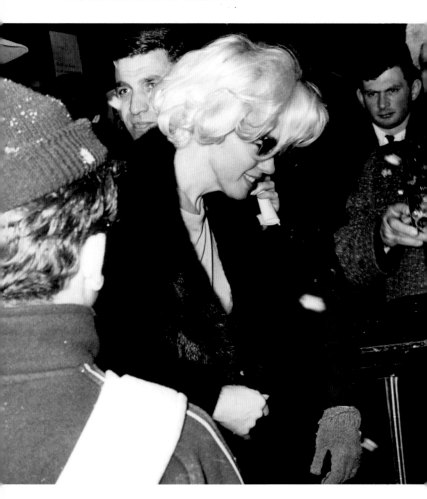

On a snowy New York evening in 1962, Marilyn makes a trip to the theater to see *Brecht on Brecht*. OPPOSITE: In February 1962, Marilyn visits Mexico to buy furnishings for her new house in Los Angeles.

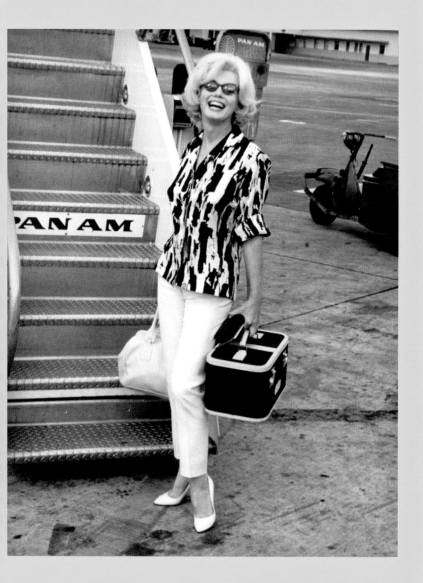

insist the star not take part in the presidential festivities. Marilyn went anyway but became ill shortly afterward, causing still more delays, and was then fired from the movie.

Her mental health and behavior on set became fodder for the tabloids, but Marilyn fought on. Her lawyers dealt with Fox, and instead of lying low, she gave numerous interviews, took part in several photo shoots, and made sure her name was kept in the headlines in a more positive light. Unfortunately, Marilyn's fragile health never improved, and she passed away on the night of August 4 or the early morning of August 5, 1962. There have been myriad speculations on the events that occurred that night, but the coroner declared her death to be a probable suicide. Her funeral was arranged by DiMaggio, and she was laid to rest at Westwood Memorial Park.

For the next twenty years, DiMaggio arranged for flowers to be delivered to Marilyn's grave, and even now—well over half a century after her death—her place of rest is never without bouquets and tributes. The constant presence of admirers at the cemetery is testimony to the fact that Marilyn is as relevant today as she was during the 1950s, and of that she would have been immensely proud.

OPPOSITE: One of the last publicity appearances Marilyn made was to sing "Happy Birthday" to President Kennedy at Madison Square Garden.

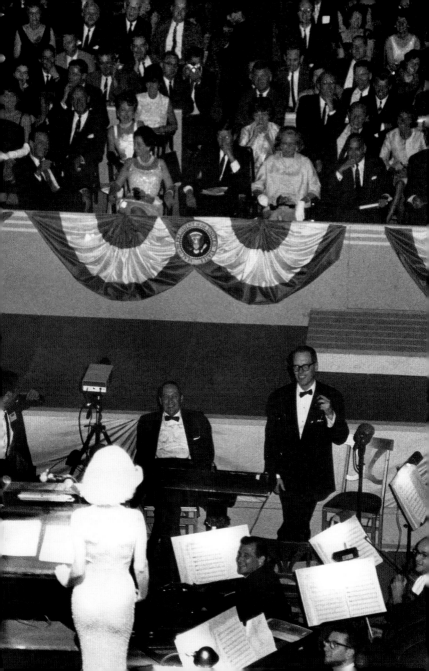

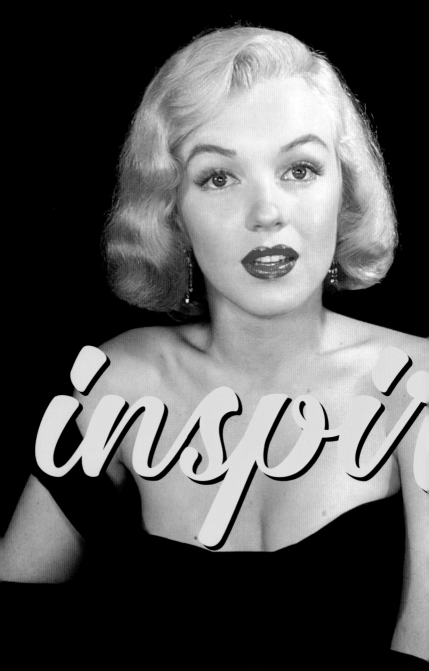

ation

AM FREQUENTLY ASKED JUST WHAT IT IS THAT KEEPS Marilyn relevant and fascinating all these years after her death. The answer is—quite literally—everything! Some people are inspired by Marilyn's fashion sense and beauty (celebrities such as Madonna, Gwen Stefani, and Anna Nicole Smith are excellent examples of this). Then there are those who love to read about her real life away from the cameras, even more who thoroughly enjoy her films, and those who ferociously collect all manner of Marilyn memorabilia. Interestingly, what first attracts us to Marilyn often evolves into something else entirely. For instance, while it was that glamorous postcard that first attracted my attention, and I still appreciate the glamour today, it is Marilyn's true personality that I am most drawn to: her inner strength, vulnerability, and determination.

As Marilyn remains ubiquitous in popular culture, it is little wonder that most of us discover her at some point in our youth. "It was 1976, and I'd just turned twelve," remembers collector Fraser Penny. "I was doing a project on famous people, and I eventually came to Marilyn and stopped. She overwhelmed me, and the project became about her alone! From then on, I started noticing her image in book shops

OPPOSITE: Marilyn during a costume test for the 1951 movie, *Love Nest*.
PREVIOUS SPREAD: An unusual publicity shot of starlet Marilyn Monroe for *The Asphalt Jungle*.

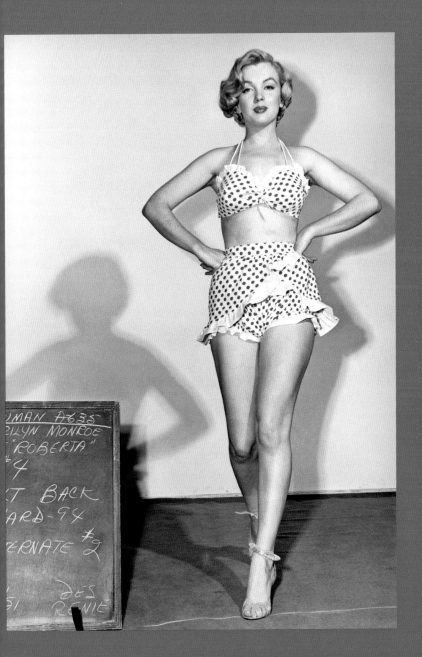

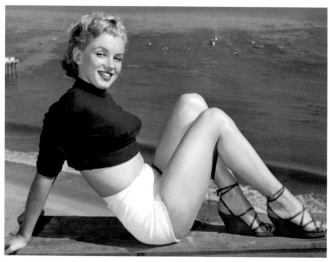

Marilyn's casual style would not look out of place today.

and pictures in newspaper and magazine articles, which I cut out and saved. When I bought the book *Norma Jean* by Fred Lawrence Guiles, the cover picture seemed to cast a spell over me, like she was looking right into my soul.

"I just collected printed items at first: books, magazines, posters, and postcards. I collected because I felt I was on a mission to preserve her memory, and if I saw something with her image, I had to have it. It was like it was made especially for me! At first it was a comfort for me to have this little collection that I could look after and add to, like a hobby. But now as an older person there's more of a fondness for

Marilyn as an enduring presence in my life. And my mother and my father are attached to many memories of watching her films together. They would buy me items to add to my collection. There is a sentimental attachment to her now. Marilyn is like a light that always shines."

Greg Schreiner became such a staunch admirer that he eventually created Marilyn Remembered, the most famous Marilyn Monroe fan club in the world: "My first introduction to Marilyn was when I was around eight years old and my parents took me to a movie drive-in located [coincidentally] in Monroe, Wisconsin. The movie was *Some Like It Hot*, and I instantly fell in love with Marilyn. She was so breathtakingly beautiful and positively glowed on the screen. I had never seen anyone like her before, and I vowed to find out more about her. Thus I started collecting whatever I could, which at that time was mostly magazines.

"I had moved to Los Angeles in 1979 to go to school at UCLA, and in 1981 I went to pay my respects at her grave. I met three other people that day: Anthony Cordova and Theresa and Catherine Seeger. We realized that nothing had been done to honor Marilyn on August 5 since her death in 1962, and we vowed to put on a small service the following year at her graveside. Because we enjoyed each other's company and sharing of Marilyn, we decided to also meet at

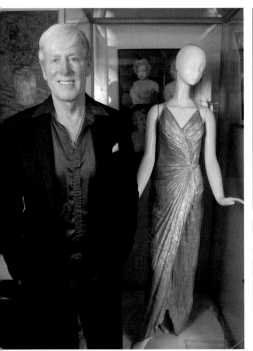

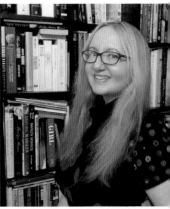

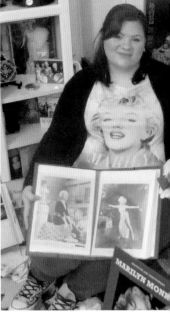

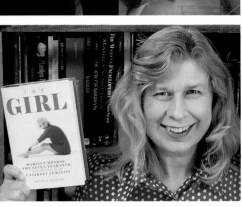

my home on a monthly basis. Thus, Marilyn Remembered was born in 1982. We have been so fortunate over the years to have incredible guest speakers, and over fifty have been people who knew Marilyn personally. The tradition continues, and we continue to meet every August 5 to provide a memorial service for fans of Ms. Monroe."

But what is it that makes Greg such a fan? "Marilyn is enduring to me because she captured my heart as a young boy and she has never left my life. I feel that many things that have occurred to me were because of Marilyn, directly or indirectly. She has enriched my life in so many ways, and I feel quite blessed. Every part of her career has inspired me—from her photos to her films and her interaction with her friends. Marilyn was adored by so many, and those who knew her are still deeply touched by her loss after all these years.

"Marilyn has inspired me to strive for what I believe in. I think the world is still fascinated by Marilyn because she was so unique and there will never be another like her. Many have tried to imitate her, and none have succeeded. She represents an incredibly loving spirit, and her inner glow shines through so clearly in both her films and photos."

OPPOSITE, CLOCKWISE FROM TOP LEFT: Greg Schreiner collects gowns and other Marilyn-related items. • Michelle Morgan has been a Marilyn fan since 1985 and has written six books about her idol, including this one! • Vanessa Roden has been inspired by Marilyn since she was a teenager. • Leslie Summey became a Marilyn fan when she was in her forties.

Johan Grimmius, an enthusiast for the past four decades, is fascinated that so many young people still know Marilyn. "It's surprising, since she died in 1962," he says. "Most stars from that time are really unknown to kids now, but not Marilyn. She is known from one generation to the next, and I think it's not only her looks that people see, it is something that people feel. That's why she still fascinates the world today—because in some way she still touches people, and that feeling can never become dated."

Megan Owen is proof of Johan's theory. "I first became a Marilyn fan in October 2010," she says. "I was almost seventeen and instantly felt fascinated and connected to her. I simply had to know more, and I bought all of her movies and lots of books and seven years on, the love just keeps on growing!

"Marilyn inspires and helps me every day. I discovered her only a few months before I began suffering from a variety of mental struggles. She has consistently helped me on my journey, and I honestly don't know who I'd be without her. In my hardest times, I often think to myself, 'If Marilyn could get through this or that, then I can do this.' To me she is definitely one of the bravest and strongest people to have lived, and I only wish she could see this for herself. She was her biggest critic.

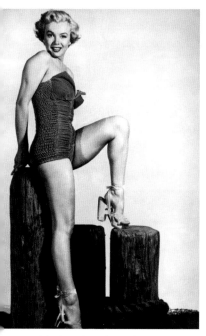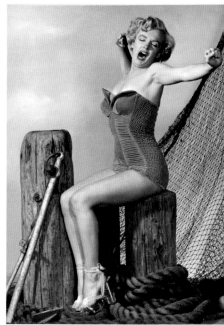

Marilyn often showed a great sense of humor in her photos, as demonstrated in these publicity shots.

"I think the world is still fascinated and inspired by Marilyn for so many reasons—her timelessness being a huge one. Throughout Hollywood there have been so many beautiful blondes, but they pale in comparison to Marilyn. She has a unique quality, she connected to her fans, and she loved and respected their belief in her. No other star has or will endure like Marilyn. Of course, many still talk about the ridiculous conspiracies, myths, and obviously her death; however, her death doesn't define her. She was so much more than what many perceive her to be."

Vanessa Roden is another who discovered Marilyn as a teenager: "I think I first became a fan when I was about eighteen years old. I'd always loved watching older movies with my grandmother, and my love seemed to grow from there. The first movie I ever saw Marilyn in was *Gentlemen Prefer Blondes*. I was completely captivated by her. Her screen presence drew me in, and I just couldn't take my eyes off of her.

"I find it difficult to explain why I like her so much, as it's a combination of things. Her personality, vulnerability, style, talent, beauty, etc. And she was such a genuine and caring person. She was just the whole package—one of a kind. I think what makes me adore her most is how she always had time for her fans. It was never too much trouble for her to sign an autograph, and she gave the public credit for making her a star.

"Marilyn always helps me when I'm feeling upset or gloomy. A simple action of putting on one of her films or watching an interview with her can bring a smile back to my face. I can't really explain why, other than she gives off a kind of warm feeling when I see her on screen. I know that she's always there for me when I need her. I also feel inspired by her to fight for what I believe in and to work hard to follow my dreams, because in Marilyn's case if you want them badly enough, they are possible."

Marisa Vanderpest has adored Marilyn for nearly thirty years. "I first became a fan of Marilyn in 1990, when I was fourteen," she says. "*Gentlemen Prefer Blondes* was on television, and my grandmother and I decided to watch it, as I knew this was the actress that Madonna had played tribute to in 'Material Girl,' and I was a huge Madonna fan. I sat in awe at Marilyn's beauty. I couldn't believe someone could be that stunning, and I still can't! She also made me laugh. Funny and beautiful—just what I wanted to be. The next day, I went to the store, where I bought my first poster and that week rented every movie my local video shop had. I was hooked. My greatest Marilyn memories are of that time, as my nana watched every one of those movies with me, and she also bought me posters and my first books.

Many fans are inspired by Marilyn because of her style.

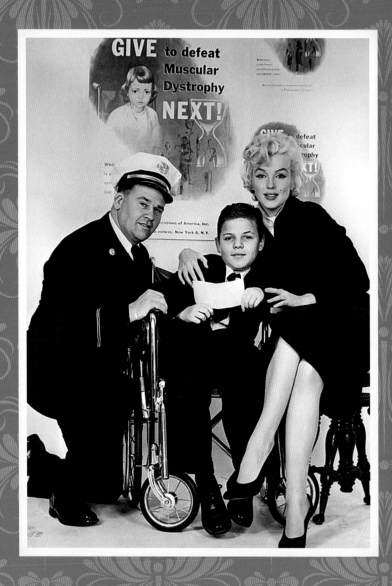

"As I got older I could afford pieces like the Franklin Mint Marilyn dolls, and then I turned to vintage items. At eighteen, I got my first old magazine with her on the cover—a 1959 issue of the Australian publication *Women's Weekly*. I love items that were produced in her lifetime that she may have seen herself. I don't have a huge collection, but I love all I own. My most cherished items are a piece of paper with her autograph and my 1952 *Golden Dreams* calendar."

While many enthusiasts come to Marilyn as teenagers, occasionally she is discovered by someone at a much older age. This is the case with Leslie Summey, who found the actress in her forties. "I'd known about Marilyn of course, since I was a child," Leslie says, "But I had never seen any of her films. It was many years later that I became drawn to her enough to find out more. Two photographs were the impetus for the discovery of my love for her. The first one I saw was at a furniture store, of all places. It was a rather ignominious beginning for an interest that would hold such a dear place in my heart and be such an important influence on my life. One day in a furniture shop I happened upon a framed wall art poster of Marilyn that I'd never seen. In fact, I wasn't even sure it was Marilyn at first because it didn't look like her. At least, it wasn't like any of

OPPOSITE: Marilyn loved helping charitable causes.

the photos I'd seen of her up to that point in my life. There was no glamorous starlet, no heavily made-up face, no fabulous gown. Instead, there was a petite, bare-footed blonde woman reclining on a work-out bench, wearing jeans and a halter top. In each hand, she gripped a free weight which she held at arm's length above her chest. I gazed at a poster-sized photo of 1950s-era Marilyn Monroe, pumping iron in a gym! I was flabbergasted. I could not stop staring at it because it was the antithesis of everything I'd ever seen of this woman. I fell in love with that picture then and there, and with its subject.

"Soon after I ran across another picture. This one was relatively famous, but still one that I'd never seen. It was by Richard Avedon and showed a pensive Marilyn. She was wearing a glamorous sequined gown with her makeup just so. To me, this was a Marilyn that was obviously a character. It was reminiscent of an old-fashioned cosplay, as if the cosplayer had been caught by the photographer just before getting into character. The look was sad, vulnerable, unsure, and filled with child-like innocence. It was not at

OPPOSITE, CLOCKWISE FROM TOP: Scott Fortner has built a magnificent collection of Marilyn's belongings. • A Marilyn doll, crocheted by doll maker Emma Mitchell. • Jessica Kiper pays tribute to Marilyn the movie star. • Marisa Vanderpest has loved Marilyn since she was fourteen years old. Two of Marisa's favorite items are replicas of Marilyn's Mexican cardigan and summer dress.

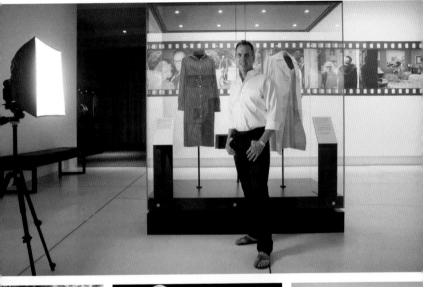

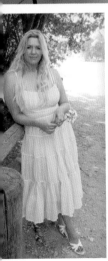

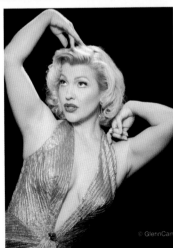

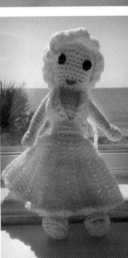

© GlennCam

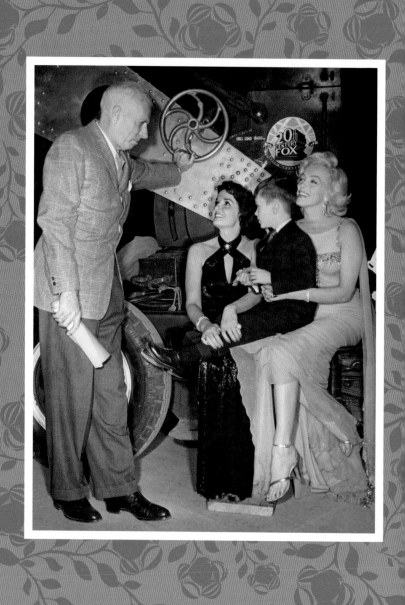

all the sexy, self-confident image of Marilyn Monroe that I had always known.

"I immediately realized that it was Norma Jeane I was seeing, and I knew then that Marilyn Monroe was only a character that she tried on when she was working. Tears sprang to my eyes, and I found myself wanting to hug her so tight . . . hug this woman who had died four years before I was even born. I felt an overwhelming need to protect her from the world. It was then I finally began to understand, on a genuine level, the real woman behind the legend and the reason why she was still just as famous nearly fifty years after her death."

For some, being inspired by Marilyn is taken to a whole new level. This is the case for Emma Mitchell, who crochets Marilyn Monroe—inspired dolls. "I think the popularity of Marilyn dolls in general is being able to have something you can hold in your hand that represents the actress. I love making them, and while it is tempting to sell the dolls, I like to keep them as a hobby, something I make because I enjoy it. My Marilyn dolls now have a far better wardrobe than me, and definitely more glamorous!"

Collector Scott Fortner does not remember the exact moment he discovered Marilyn, but her influence on his life

OPPOSITE: Marilyn and Jane Russell relax on the set of *Gentlemen Prefer Blondes*.

has been monumental. When asked what made the actress such an enduring figure for him, he answered: "I was asked a similar question during the opening of one of my exhibits in Australia in 2016. My response was, 'You don't pick Marilyn; Marilyn picks you.' From that angle and perspective, it's really impossible to articulate or even understand what makes her such an enduring figure for me. We all have individual mental and emotional connections to various elements in our world. For nearly forty years now, for me it's been Marilyn Monroe. She'll always be part of my life, and I barely recall a time when she wasn't.

"Marilyn was quite accomplished. I wouldn't say she inspires me, but she definitely impresses me. Her achievements are miraculous, considering her shaky upbringing and limited formal education. She became a sought-after model and a major film star, she married not one but two incredibly accomplished men, and she overcame obstacles and experienced great success. She pulled away from the studio system in the mid-1950s in a way other stars wouldn't dare, and she opened her own production company. She never received recognition in the US for her more serious film roles, but both France and Italy recognized her with their highest honors for her acting abilities. She met the queen of England, the president of the United States, and other world leaders. Not bad for a pinup girl!"

For many, discovering Marilyn has literally changed their lives. Jessica "Sugar" Kiper, aka tribute artist Amer-Icon Monroe, is a fine example of that. "I have been inspired by Marilyn since I was twelve years old. A few people had told me that I looked like her, and when I watched *Some Like It Hot* with my father, I couldn't believe anyone saw a little bit of this glamorous movie star in *me*! That summer, I lightened my hair, and when I went back to school, the pretty, popular girls started picking on me, but I had confidence for once, so I tried not to let them get me down. I've since done the things I proclaimed I would do, such as in class when they asked us what we would like to do one day, I said, 'Modeling and acting.' I've also received an apology from the main mean girl, after she saw me in a television show. It was healing for my inner child. Marilyn changed my life that summer, and she literally shaped who I am today. I hope somehow she knows how loved she is even to this day, by so many around the world."

chapter

THREE

style

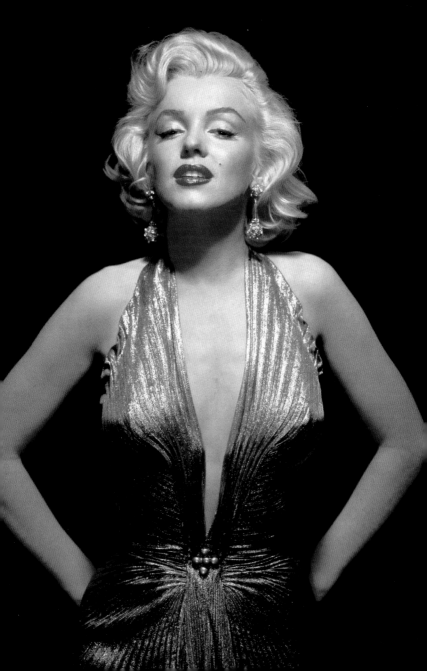

❝ WISH A GOOD STYLIST WOULD TAKE OVER MARILYN Monroe's clothes problem. It's hard for a girl with that gorgeous figure to go so wrong on clothes—but Marilyn accomplishes it." So wrote acerbic columnist Louella Parsons in 1952. Louella was actually quite a champion of Marilyn's career, but her thoughts on her attire are revealing. The fact is that while young women today see Marilyn as a fashionable figure, many in the 1950s did not appreciate her clothes at all.

It would be fair to say that Marilyn's style was eclectic. Her public persona was sexy and glamorous, with wonderfully tight gowns that emphasized every curve. This was hard for the old-school Hollywood elite to understand or accept. However, what they perhaps didn't realize was that Marilyn owned very few gowns of her own, and for public events, she frequently raided the costume department at Twentieth Century Fox. Therefore, the style that so enraged bitter movie queens and columnists alike was not actually Marilyn's at all, but the studio's.

In private, Marilyn wore casual and modern clothes, such as pants, blouses, cardigans, and sweaters. Indeed, one of her most famous outfits was the Mexican cardigan used for a beach shoot with photographer George Barris, just months before she passed away. It is frequently said that

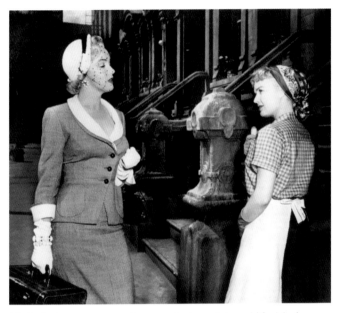

Marilyn's characters were often smartly dressed. In real life, Marilyn preferred simple shirts and slacks.

one could pick up the actress from the 1950s and drop her straight into 2018, and nobody would think her clothes odd or old-fashioned. Most of the style of items she wore during her days off are still widely available across the world.

While it is fun to admire the glamorous gowns of Hollywood's yesterday, parading around in taffeta and velvet is not something we tend to do very often. Therefore, in this section we will mainly concentrate on Marilyn's own private wardrobe, rather than the costumes she wore in movies and at film premieres.

One of the most common remarks I hear after telling someone I'm a Marilyn fan is, "But you don't look like her at all!" I used to be flabbergasted and confused by such a statement, but perhaps I shouldn't have been. After all, while most of us do not resemble Marilyn, many do enjoy collecting her style of clothing. Those lucky enough to share her qualities even take the interest further by adopting not only Marilyn's fashion but her hair, makeup, and accessories, too.

"Marilyn's style most definitely inspires my own," says Megan Owen. "Without doubt, I feel I'm a vintage girl at heart. I live in 1950s dresses, anything floral, fitted, and sweetheart neck-lined. I actually can't remember the last time I wore pants. Every day is a dress day! I also love to pin-curl my hair, and my makeup is similar to Marilyn's—red lipstick and winged eyeliner is a must. Marilyn's most iconic dresses are probably the white one from *The Seven Year Itch*, the pink from her 'Diamonds Are a Girl's Best Friend' musical number, and the one she wore to sing

OPPOSITE, CLOCKWISE FROM TOP LEFT: Megan Owen is inspired by 1950s fashions. • Adopting Marilyn's style has made Kaylie Minzola feel more confident. • Kaity Kinloch dresses in Marilyn's style when working and in everyday life. • Lookalike Blonde Fox loves performing as Marilyn.

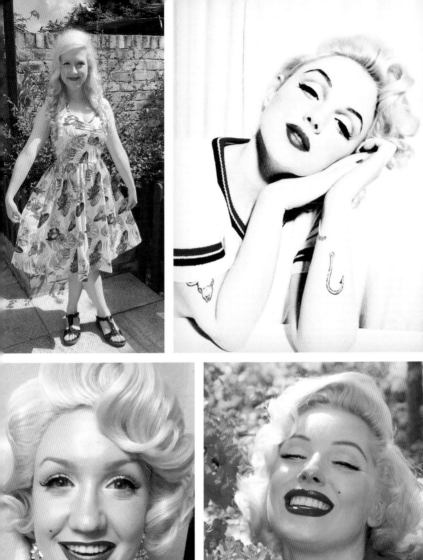
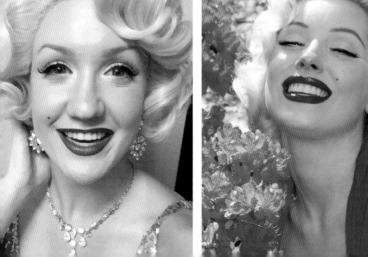

'Happy Birthday' to JFK. However, once you discover Marilyn's whole style across her thirty-six years, you will find there are so many other amazing options; it's not always about the obvious choices."

Kaylie Minzola finds that dressing in a Marilyn-inspired way has a surprising effect on people. "I get a lot of positive reactions," she says. "Sometimes people will ask for a photo with me. I find that older people and young women are the most excited about my appearance, and I get a lot of questions about my hair and makeup. Most men my age (early twenties) actually find it a little off-putting and odd. Oh well! When I'm dressed like Marilyn, I can't help but feel more confident. Adopting her style has helped me feel more comfortable with myself, while still maintaining my individuality. Marilyn has helped me stand out a little more, and break away from some social anxiety I used to feel. Since people come up and talk to me or ask me questions, she has helped me come out of my shell. I like to help keep Marilyn's memory alive by dressing the part!"

Kaity Kinloch is a tribute artist known as Marilyn Performs, and her job resulted after admiring Marilyn for many years. "I used to look at pictures of her when I was a teenager," she says, "and I was in awe of her beauty. When I was older and researched her life story, my admiration remained, but instead of finding value in her appearance, I found myself being able to deeply relate to her and her outlook on life, which was much more valuable to me. Her outward beauty became somewhat second best in comparison to the new appeal I found in her beautiful soul.

"I am not happy in a lot of frills and furbelows, so I find it always turns out for the best to follow my own ideas about my clothes."—MARILYN

"My appreciation for Marilyn really doesn't start and stop with each performance. I dress in her style in my everyday life, which, as you can probably imagine, garners a lot of attention. I feel as though Marilyn's legacy is skewed and distorted, and many people hold ignorant and shameful opinions of her. I get a lot of questions daily, and really I don't mind. I enjoy informing people of what I know about Marilyn, and they usually appreciate the truth, instead of these strange misconceptions about her."

A tribute artist known as Blonde Fox Entertainment loves the effect dressing like Marilyn has on people. "There are so many amazing experiences that have happened while performing as Marilyn. I once saw a veteran who had met her, and he was so excited that I was there. We brought him back for a special photo opportunity, and I sang songs just for him. I love seeing people's faces light up when I walk on stage, and they say, 'She looks just like her,' or 'She sounds just like her,' or they know immediately before I have done anything who I am. Marilyn was always the brightest light in a room, and to be able to emulate that light and that energy is amazing."

Marilyn's clothes are a great source of self-assurance and cheer to many women around the world. Lookalike Ashley Clark explains how dressing like the star helped her overcome bullying:

"I think I found myself wearing 'homage' fashion more often than my usual attire because at the time, I wasn't happy with how I was being seen and interpreted by my peers—I was bullied and still recovering from that part of my life. I felt comfort in hiding myself behind theatrical roles. Selecting a Marilyn-esque top or skirt was a great relief, because I almost didn't feel responsible for it! It was a fashion choice made by an icon. I could vicariously stand behind her style choices with confidence, and if anyone were to say anything about it, I could brush it off much easier than if it had been directed at just me. Marilyn's clothing taste was

OPPOSITE: Young Marilyn wears a sensible outfit to meet the mayor of Los Angeles, Fletcher Bowron.

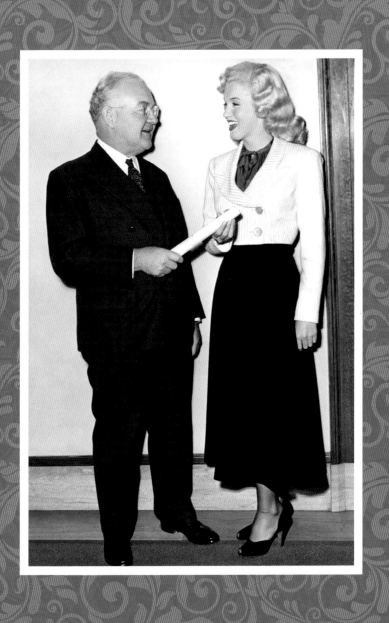

like a shield, which is ironic, as she once said people would be aggressive to her—as if there wasn't a real flesh-and-blood person in front of them—or, as she phrased it, 'as if it were happening to your clothes.' Well for me, it was!"

"My main advice to all girls seeking glamour is very simple—be yourself! Glamour is not all low-cut gowns and the slinky look. Blue jeans and overalls can still make you look attractive, if you follow a few simple hints."—MARILYN

Actress and tribute artist Hanna Nixon takes Marilyn's fashions seriously: "I was twelve years old when I first discovered her in a calendar on my brother's bedroom wall, and I turn thirty-seven this year. I am influenced mostly by Marilyn's daily life rather than the showbiz icon we have all come to recognize. For me, the items she chose for her personal wardrobe speak more about her than the glamorous gowns—her bright Pucci blouses, plain jersey dresses, Mexican sweaters, and of course her checked pants. When

OPPOSITE, TOP AND LOWER RIGHT: Mariam Myrone's hobby is to make replicas of Marilyn's clothes. LOWER LEFT: Laura Kallio models a Marilyn-inspired dress made by Esther Smith.

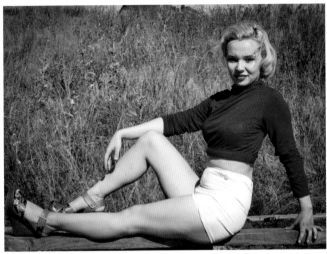

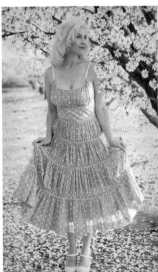

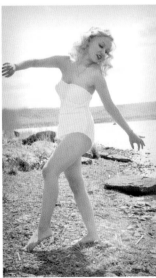

trying to work out exactly what it is about Marilyn that influences me, I struggle. It's not just one thing, it's many: her style—ever current and timeless; her elegance—even in jeans—and her uniqueness."

Some people enjoy making replicas of Marilyn's clothes, both as a business and for fun. Mariam Myrone does not sell her pieces but instead poses in them for her Instagram posts. "I never dress like Marilyn for public events," she says. "It is just my big hobby. Most of Marilyn's outfits look up-to-date enough so they can be worn in our modern society, and of course her style is feminine. All of her wardrobe was tailored to her figure and perfectly emphasized her charming body. Every girl wants to be beautiful and desired. There is nothing wrong with being fashionable and on trend, but if you want to stand out from the crowd, then Marilyn's style is just what you need."

Dress designers Allyson Scanlon and Esther Smith both make replica clothes and outfits for others to enjoy. "Whether you are a young teenager or an older, mature woman, Marilyn's style has appeal, is sexy without looking tarty, and is still fashionable today," says Allyson. "I wanted to make copies of her dresses in comfortable, stretchy fabrics such as Lycra and jersey, so that they could be worn every day. The leopard muff and cape are very popular. They

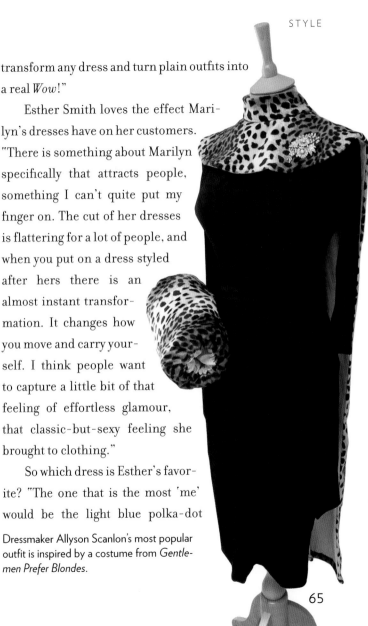

transform any dress and turn plain outfits into a real *Wow!*"

Esther Smith loves the effect Marilyn's dresses have on her customers. "There is something about Marilyn specifically that attracts people, something I can't quite put my finger on. The cut of her dresses is flattering for a lot of people, and when you put on a dress styled after hers there is an almost instant transformation. It changes how you move and carry yourself. I think people want to capture a little bit of that feeling of effortless glamour, that classic-but-sexy feeling she brought to clothing."

So which dress is Esther's favorite? "The one that is the most 'me' would be the light blue polka-dot

Dressmaker Allyson Scanlon's most popular outfit is inspired by a costume from *Gentlemen Prefer Blondes*.

dress with all the ruffles and piping. It's not my favorite dress to make. I'm not a big fan of sewing ruffles, but it is sweet and relaxed, not as obviously sexy as some of the others.

"I won't be satisfied until people want to hear me sing without looking at me. Of course that doesn't mean I want them to stop looking." —MARILYN

"People often tell me they have a wedding, vacation, party, or convention coming up, and it's a 'great excuse to have something made.' I have received great feedback from customers over the years, and the most popular is 'This makes me feel like Marilyn.' I never get tired of hearing that, but when someone writes, 'I was crying putting this dress on. . . . It fits perfectly, and I felt beautiful for the first time in a long time,' that really is my favorite part of what I do. Knowing I've helped make someone feel good about themselves makes my day."

Fans are not the only ones inspired by Marilyn. In 2009, Dolce & Gabbana showcased dresses printed with Marilyn's face for their fall collection. Then in the same year, Scarlett

Johansson was photographed à la Marilyn to advertise Dolce & Gabbana's cosmetics campaign.

In 2011, Dior chose Marilyn and Grace Kelly to help actress Charlize Theron advertise J'Adore perfume. The televised commercial used a CGI version of the actress holding a bottle of the scent. Two years later, Chanel revealed that Marilyn would be the face of Chanel No. 5 and used archive footage and photographs in the campaign.

Also in 2013, Macy's department store announced a Marilyn-inspired collection, which included summer dresses in white, stripes, and red gingham; denim shorts; a shirt tied at the waist; and a striped pencil skirt. This is not the only time the star has been used as a muse for such collections. A year earlier, an official brand of jewelry was released, and world-famous Marilyn look-alike Suzie Kennedy was chosen to front the publicity campaign.

Perhaps the most famous use of Marilyn's image by a designer came in 1991, when Versace used the Andy Warhol pop-art print on a dress modeled by Naomi Campbell. In 2017, Donatella Versace paid tribute to her brother Gianni by revisiting the idea for the company's spring 2018 collection. Fashionistas were thrilled to find that this time Marilyn's image was used not only on a dress but on boots, tights, and a shirt, too.

CREATING YOUR WARDROBE

BULLET BRAS AND BUSTIERS

During the 1950s, Marilyn was rumored to wear no underwear at all. However, recent auctions confirm that she certainly owned her fair share of bras and bustiers. In her early days as a "sweater girl," it is evident that Norma Jeane wore a bullet bra underneath her clothes. Popular during the 1950s for making a woman's chest resemble two pyramids, the bullet bra has not stood the test of time but can still be found in vintage-inspired shops and online. However, a cheaper option is a seamed bra (identifiable by the seams running horizontally and vertically across the garment), which is still widely available in modern fashion stores.

Almost as soon as her pinup days were over, Marilyn preferred a softer, more feminine look. Billy Wilder, director of *The Seven Year Itch*, remembered that she once appeared on set with what seemed to be a bra underneath her nightdress. When the director commented on it, the actress told him that she was not wearing any undergarments at all and that her breasts were unsupported. Mar-

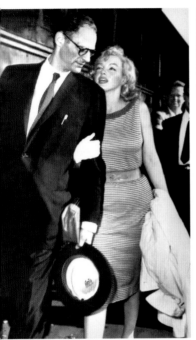 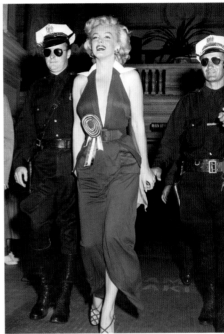

FROM LEFT: Marilyn often wore jersey dresses. • Marilyn caused a sensation in this low-cut number during a publicity event in Atlantic City.

ilyn may have been lucky enough to need no support, but the rest of us likely do. In that regard, it is good to take inspiration from the items sold at the Christie's estate auction in 1999. These bustiers show that Marilyn wore a rounded, padded cup in sizes 36B and 36C, in black and cream. While these garments may not be as popular today as in previous years, bustiers are still widely available at retailers such as Victoria's Secret and What Katie Did.

PENCIL SKIRTS

There seemed to be two types of women during the 1950s: those who enjoyed wearing swing or pleated skirts and dresses, and those who preferred the more sophisticated line of the pencil (called such because of its straight cut). While Marilyn was occasionally seen wearing a swing or pleat, she was more a fan of pencils and wore them throughout the 1950s and into the '60s. Neutral colors were often chosen for skirts and then teamed with a sweater or plain shirt. The dresses were sometimes more colorful and came in a variety of shades, such as hot pink. Some were even striped or checked and then belted for definition at the waist.

Thanks to the continuing popularity of pencil skirts and "wiggle" dresses, they can still be found in most women's clothing stores. More vintage-inspired ones are also available from online shops such as Glamour Bunny, Pinup Girl Clothing, Collectif, and Stop Staring!

OPPOSITE: During the making of *Niagara* in 1952, Marilyn often borrowed the costumes to wear off the set.

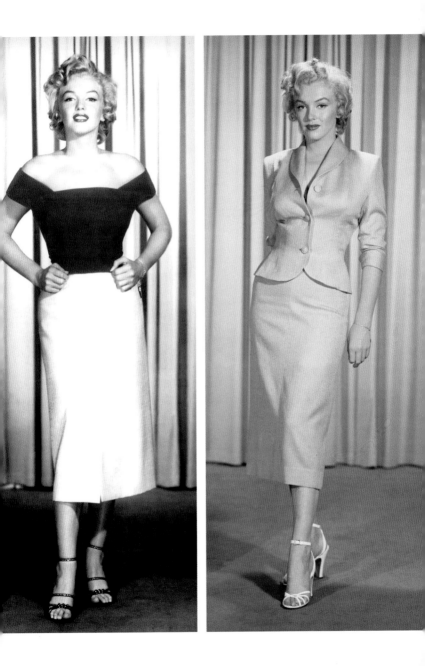

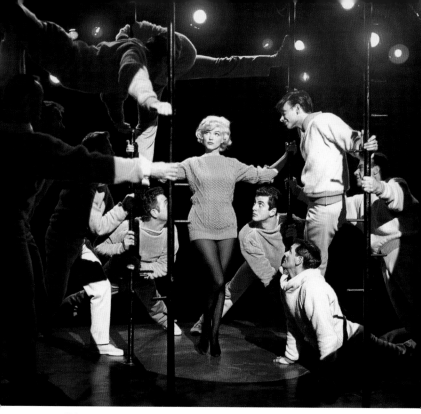

Wearing a sweater on the set of *Let's Make Love* in 1960.

SWEATERS AND CARDIGANS

Marilyn's relationship with sweaters and cardigans was long and passionate. Thanks to the sweater she was photographed in by David Conover in 1945, and the famous Mexican cardigan that featured in beach photos by George Barris in 1962, you could say that knitwear truly framed Marilyn's career.

Short and mid-length sweaters were most popular, especially during her New York days in the mid-1950s, but she was also occasionally photographed wearing a longer design—the most famous perhaps being the red one used in a Milton Greene shoot. Another instance of wearing knitwear happened during a trip to England in 1956. Marilyn was spotted riding her bike in Windsor Great Park while wearing a loose cardigan and pants. Of course a photographer was there to record the event, and the photos were beamed around the world.

As with the pencil skirt, sweaters and cardigans are among those classic lines that have never gone out of fashion. The Gap sells a host of 1950s knitwear, and several years ago it even stocked a Mexican-style cardigan. The item was first spotted in a small store in England, and the news brought hysteria to the Marilyn community, with customers around the globe clamoring to buy one. Pinup Girl Clothing also stocks 1950s sweaters in a variety of colors.

JEANS

Marilyn was a trailblazer in most areas of her life, and this trickled down into her wardrobe, too. While it was mainly men who wore jeans in the 1950s, Marilyn was often spotted in the garments both on and off-screen. "I buy boy's jeans

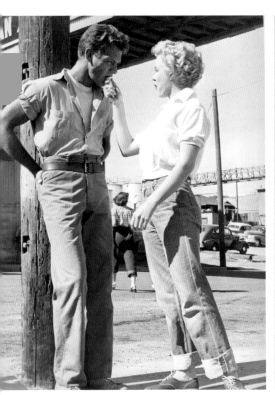

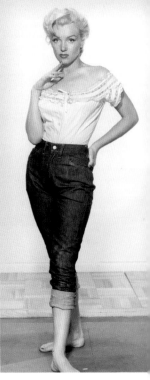

FROM LEFT: Marilyn wears jeans in the 1952 movie *Clash by Night*, and the 1954 film *River of No Return*.

because they're long-waisted like me," she said. While a model during the mid-1940s, she was photographed by André de Dienes in flared jeans with huge cuffs. Her taste changed to slim-fitted jeans during the 1950s, as she explained to *Photoplay* magazine: "I have always felt comfortable in blue jeans; they're my favorite informal attire. I have to admit that I like mine to fit. There's nothing I hate worse than baggy blue jeans." Early in her career, Marilyn was photographed jogging the back streets of Beverly Hills in her high-waisted jeans and spent a considerable amount of time wearing denim in 1952's *Clash by Night*. They also formed a large part of *The Misfits* wardrobe in 1960. Whether straight-legged, flared, or high-waisted, jeans are a staple part of your Marilyn wardrobe—and don't forget to turn up the cuffs!

CAPRI PANTS

Other items that proved popular in Marilyn's wardrobe— particularly from the mid-1950s onward—were mid- length (or capri) pants. Tight-legged and in all manner of colors and designs, Marilyn wore these trousers mainly in casual situations: at the Actors Studio, around the house, for a walk on the beach, playing summer sports, or gardening at her Fifth Helena Drive home. Worn in colors and designs including orange, pink, white, striped, and checked, these pants can be found almost everywhere, including supermarkets and chains. However, if it's a specific vintage appearance you're after, stores such as Glamour Bunny, Pinup Girl Clothing, and Lindy Bop also stock them.

CHECKED PANTS

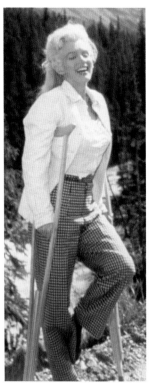

If there is one item guaranteed to work Marilyn enthusiasts into a frenzy, it is the checked (or dogtooth) pants that she was photographed in through-out her entire career. From the high-waisted flares used in early modeling shoots, through to the mid-length turnups she loved to wear on her days off, checks played an important part in Marilyn's wardrobe. Today the fashion is quite widely available.

Marilyn loved checked pants, and they remain extremely popular with fans.

BLOUSES

When Marilyn wasn't wearing a sweater, her skirts or pants would be accompanied by an elegant shirt. She wore classic short-sleeved, buttoned blouses in creams, whites, and blacks; depending on the weather she could tie them at the front to reveal a glimpse of midriff. Longer shirts sported three-quarter-length sleeves and were worn unbuttoned at the neck. On casual days, Marilyn would often wear her hair unstyled, with just a touch of makeup (or even just a layer of moisturizer) on her face. Thanks to the everlasting appeal of such items, 1950s shirts are still available almost everywhere, including The Gap and other retailers.

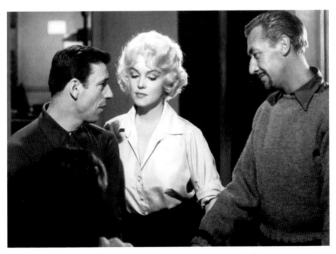

Marilyn on the set of *Let's Make Love*, wearing a casual shirt.

SWIMWEAR

In the early days of her career, Marilyn frequently wore swimwear as part of her modeling and pinup work. Most bikinis would comprise high-waist bottoms or shorts with a full bra top. However, some were a little more elaborate and included ruffles, lace, polka dots, and even bows. One bikini was made from a fishnet material, though it was lined to avoid any wardrobe malfunctions.

Perhaps the most scandalous of all Marilyn's early pinup two-piece suits was olive green with a darker green stripe. The top was strapless and tied in front with string. The bottoms were cut low at the waist and included ruffles at the top of the thighs and string at the sides.

Full swimsuits often included a sweetheart neckline and were strapless or had a halter neck. All were typically 1950s, with elastic panels to emphasize the figure and cut modestly at the thighs. Throughout the early 1950s, Marilyn was photographed in a variety of bright, bold colors, including gold, yellow, blue, and red. These suits were often worn with her favorite Lucite shoes or strapped sandals.

Marilyn-style swimwear is occasionally available in women's dress stores, but for a wider selection, it's best to check online. The official Esther Williams website has many different styles to choose from, as does Bettylicious.

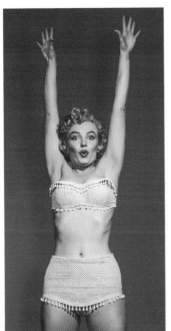

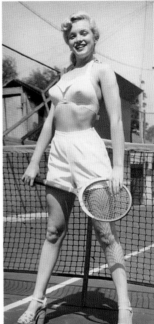

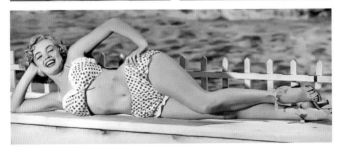

CLOCKWISE FROM TOP LEFT: This unusual bikini was made from a fishnet material and included tassels.• High-waisted shorts, a bikini top, and cork sandals are ideal for a pretend game of tennis! • Polka dots were popular on bikinis, dresses, and even gloves.

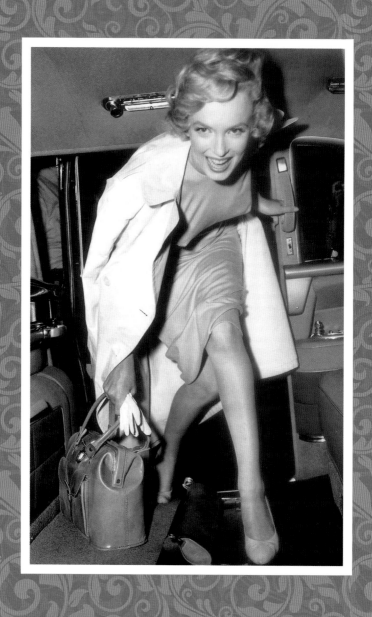

HANDBAGS

When Marilyn's belongings were sold in 1999, several handbags were featured in the auction catalog. Among them were a red satin bag from Saks Fifth Avenue, a green silk bag with a short strap, and an orange satin clutch. These elegant but simple designs were used frequently by the actress when she was at parties or premieres. An exception came when Marilyn placed her hand and footprints into cement at Grauman's Chinese Theatre in 1953. On this occasion, she opted for a small basket with a lid, which looked rather like one you'd expect to see filled with sewing supplies.

While Marilyn favored small clutch bags for parties and premieres, she opted for large leather handbags whenever she traveled or made a movie. These fashion items accommodated her script, personal items, and of course, a good book.

Perhaps the best-known of all of Marilyn's handbags is the Lucite bag she used in the 1953 movie *Niagara*. This beautifully designed, clear-colored piece was rectangular in shape, with a curved handle. It featured in much of the movie, including the famous scene where Marilyn walks away from the camera. Although finding one exactly the same as Marilyn's is quite a task, Lucite bags can still be

OPPOSITE: Marilyn's everyday handbags were often large enough to hold several books.

found on auction sites such as eBay and at antique fairs and stores. Beware though, as the delicate nature of the material causes them to deteriorate over time, and once the material starts to breakdown, there is little you can do to stop it.

HATS

Marilyn's film roles sometimes required her to wear fancy hats with feathers, veils, and fur. In real life, however, the actress wore head scarves in various colors and designs, berets in cream and black, large felt hats in various colors, and straw hats. The casual straw look was especially popular with her during the Arthur Miller years and beyond, when she spent a lot of time working in the garden. Her straw hats came in several different styles and colors. One popular design was black, with a pointed crown and wide brim. Some were 1930s in design, with huge, floppy brims. Others were smaller and included flower decorations around the crown.

Authentic 1950s hats can still be found in antique stores. However, for those wishing to buy new, most designs have been reproduced over the years in items available today.

OPPOSITE, FROM LEFT: Marilyn wears a beret on the set of *Gentlemen Prefer Blondes*.• Marilyn wears an unusual hat while on holiday in Jamaica, January 1957. • Marilyn in a beautiful straw hat and denim jacket on the set of *The Misfits*.

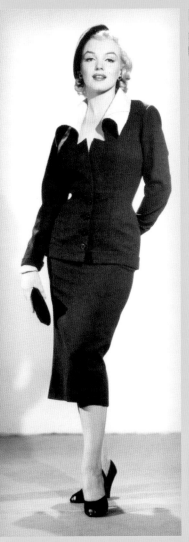
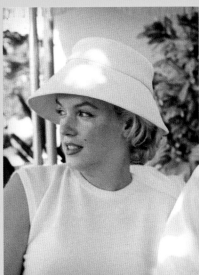
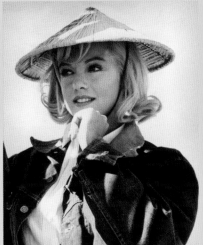

SHOES

Marilyn Monroe had many pairs of shoes in her wardrobe, from sandals to winter boots and everything in between. High-heeled pumps were immensely popular for work, shopping, and going to acting class. Favorite colors included black, white, and cream, though she also owned red, gold, blue, and even polka-dot pairs. Strapped sandals were also a popular choice, and a particular gold pair was worn frequently, including in early publicity photos and even during

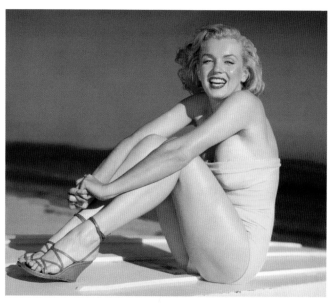

Marilyn often recycled shoes and sandals. These were seen on many occasions, throughout her early career.

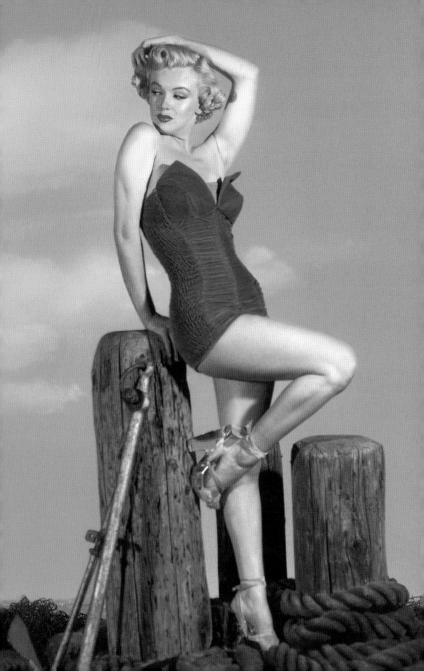

a trip to Korea to entertain the troops. In other pinup shots, Marilyn sported a pair of canvas sandals with a cork sole. These summer classics have never really gone out of fashion.

In swimwear publicity photographs taken in the early 1950s, Marilyn often wore a beautiful pair of high-heeled Lucite sandals. These creations were ingenious because the straps were actually interchangeable ribbons. This meant that whatever color swimsuit Marilyn was wearing, the same colored ribbon could be applied to the sandals. This gave the impression that she was wearing different shoes each time, though in reality, Marilyn was recycling the same pair.

One of Marilyn's favorite shoe designers was Salvatore Ferragamo. However, during her time in London, Marilyn discovered another manufacturer: Anello & Davide. Made to the actress's exact measurements, a pair of red platform sandals was worn to a performance of Arthur Miller's play, *A View from the Bridge*, while a gold pair was revealed when Marilyn met Queen Elizabeth. Marilyn loved the shoes made for her by Anello & Davide, and they remained in her collection for the rest of her life. It seems that the admiration was mutual, and a signed photograph of the star is currently displayed on the company's website.

OPPOSITE: While meeting the queen of England, Marilyn wore a stunning pair of platform sandals.

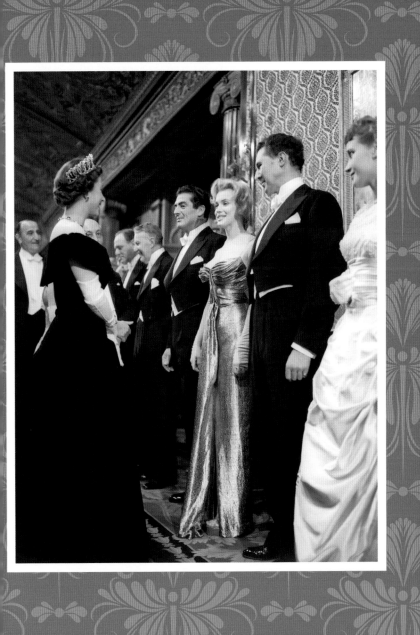

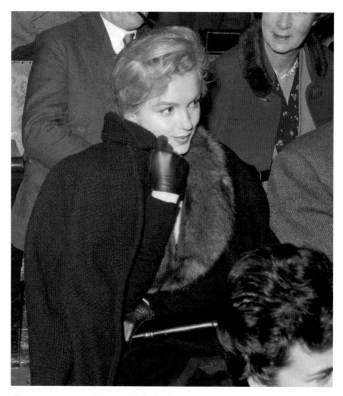

Gloves were a staple part of Marilyn's wardrobe, off-screen and on.

GLOVES

While we wear gloves or mittens to protect our hands in winter, modern women don't often have the opportunity of wearing them as dress accessories, unless they happen to be movie stars. Marilyn was a true fan of gloves and wore them regularly when she was at public events. Her collection was vast and included elbow-length pairs in black, cream, red, purple, and white; short styles in beige and black; and even a crocheted pair in black. Materials included satin, suede, nylon, and silk.

Fancy gloves are no longer a regular sight, but they can still be found in select stores. If you want to feel like a princess, however, check out British manufacturer Cornelia James. The company has been making gloves for the queen since 1947, and it offers international shipping.

JEWELRY

Despite singing "Diamonds Are a Girl's Best Friend," Marilyn did not wear a lot of jewelry herself, and most of what she did own was costume, not real. When attending a film premiere or party, the actress would often wear large, dangling rhinestone earrings with lots of sparkle and glamour. Imitation pearl earrings were popular for more serious events, such as interviews or press conferences, while in private her ears were usually bare. But no matter what earrings she wore, they would always be clip-ons, as Marilyn did not have pierced ears.

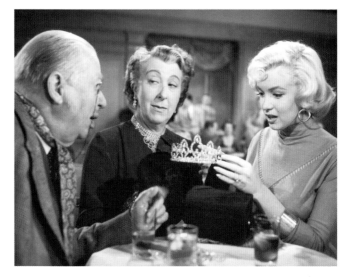

Marilyn wasn't a huge fan of jewelry, but Lorelei Lee, Marilyn's character in *Gentlemen Prefer Blondes*, loved it!

For the most part, Marilyn sported a bare neck, but if she did wear a necklace, it would often be in the form of costume beads, pearls, or crystals. Rhinestone brooches were a popular choice for jackets or dresses, and although she occasionally wore a watch or bracelet, rings were quite a rarity. Even when she was married, Marilyn didn't always wear her wedding ring.

Thanks to flea markets and antique stores, vintage costume jewelry is still extremely easy to find, and there are many bargains to be had for those willing to search through piles of jewels. Look out for auction catalogs, too. They often sell many pieces together in one lot, at relatively cheap prices.

PUCCI

While plain shirts were immensely popular throughout the 1950s, toward the end of her life Marilyn began wearing Emilio Pucci designs regularly. When her belongings went for auction at Christie's in 1999, the sheer amount of Pucci shirts and dresses was mind-blowing. Featuring colors such as orange, deep and pale pink, blue, and lime, the outfits were often long-sleeved, boat-necked, and accompanied—where applicable—by a fabric belt. Long-sleeved buttoned shirts were also popular, with bold colors, textures, and fabrics.

One tribute artist who loves Pucci is Kaity Kinloch. "In my opinion, Marilyn was an early 1960s trendsetter with her love of Pucci's bright and colorful jersey-knit fashions. Marilyn was ahead of the fashion game, and I have no doubt that this would have continued into the decade if her life story didn't end so abruptly."

Perhaps the reason so many of us think about Marilyn in Pucci (especially when we imagine her in the Fifth

Helena Drive home), is because of photographs published in the weeks leading up to her death. Scott Fortner runs the Marilyn Monroe Collection website and is lucky enough to have bought Marilyn's lime green Pucci shirt at auction. For those who cannot afford Marilyn's actual clothing but would still like a real taste of Pucci, outfits can be bought directly from the company itself. Comfortingly, the modern designs still sport fabrics and patterns remarkably like the ones Marilyn herself wore in the 1960s. And if your budget doesn't quite stretch to an authentic Pucci design, you'll be relieved to know that items inspired by the colors and lines of the 1960s garments are often spotted in modern-day stores.

Luckily, the same is true for much of Marilyn's wardrobe. "I've found outfits all over the place through the years," says Monroe student Rebecca Swift. "Once the internet arrived, it was easy. There are so many places now to buy vintage clothes and accessories. There are also clothing lines that only produce vintage-look clothes, such as Lindy Bop or Hell Bunny, and I can get lost on their websites! And of course eBay has been a massive tool for finding items. When I was a teenager, I used to get a lot from charity shops or second-hand stores, and antique fairs and centers have always been good for sourcing jewelry and accessories.

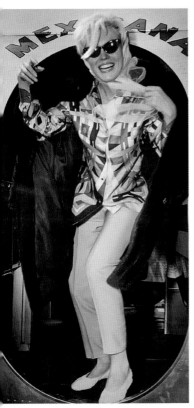
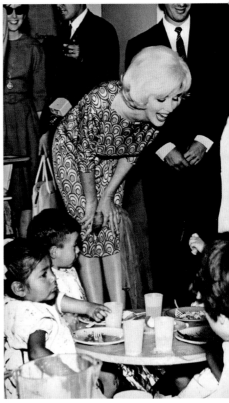

In the last two years of Marilyn's life, she was a huge fan of brightly colored outfits such as those by the designer Emilio Pucci.

It's always nice when you find something brand new that has a vintage influence. Many shops now seem to carry items that have a retro feel."

MAKE YOUR OWN DRAWSTRING PURSE

During the making of *Bus Stop*, Milton Greene took a great many photographs of Marilyn dressed as Cherie, her character in the movie. One of the props she used was a pretty drawstring bag, which has inspired the purse in the following tutorial.

Note: In this lesson we have used green fabric and ribbon with a black lace trim because that matches the one Marilyn used in the photo shoot. However, you can use any color you wish. Our finished bag measures approximately 10 inches from top to bottom, but if you want a different size purse, just change the measurements accordingly.

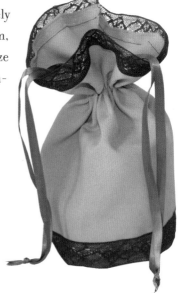

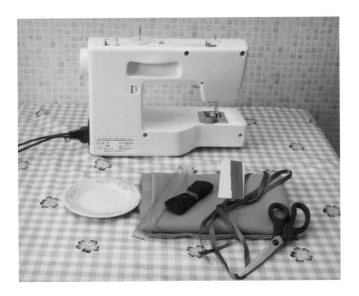

WHAT YOU WILL NEED:

- ○ medium-thickness fabric, approximately 12 inches by 45 inches

- ○ 40 inches of lace, about 1 inch wide

- ○ approximately 60 inches of medium ribbon

- ○ dressmaker's pins

- ○ small safety pin

- ○ bias binding, approximately 20 inches

- ○ thread

- ○ scissors

- ○ saucer or small bowl

- ○ ruler or tape measure

- ○ tailor's chalk or pencil

- ○ sewing machine (optional)

95

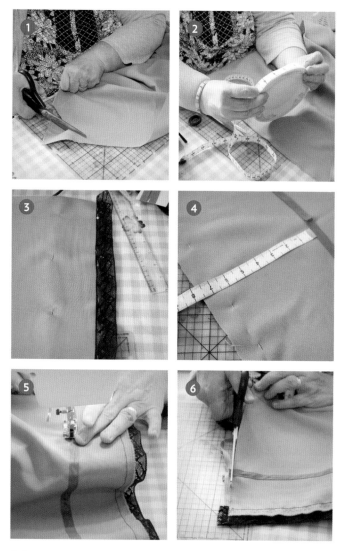

1) Carefully draw a circle at the edge of your material, using a saucer or small bowl. We used tailor's chalk to do this, but a pencil or pen will work just as well. Then cut the circle out.

2) Measure the circumference of the saucer or bowl to give an estimate of how much material you need to cut out for the body of the bag. Ours measured 20 inches, and we allowed 1/2 inch for the seam. Cut the material out, and then using the same circumference measurements, cut two pieces of lace and one of bias binding.

3) With the material facing right side up, pin one of the lace pieces along the bottom edge of the material. Then the second piece of lace should be pinned at the top of the material, on the neatened or hemmed edge. Allow it to hang above the top of the fabric by about 1/2 inch.

4) On the other side of the fabric, pin the bias binding, approximately 7-1/2 inches from the bottom. You will need the ruler or tape measure at this point, to make sure the binding is straight all the way along.

5) Either with a sewing machine or by hand, attach the two pieces of lace onto the fabric. Then run a row of stitches at the top of the bias binding and another at the bottom, as close to the edges as possible. This creates a channel for the ribbon to pass through later.

6) Trim off any loose threads, and then fold the fabric in half, making sure that the bias binding is facing upward. Pin in place and then sew the two edges together, stopping about an inch from the bottom, so that the lace does not get stitched into the seam. Optional: if you'd like to make sure the edges don't fray, you

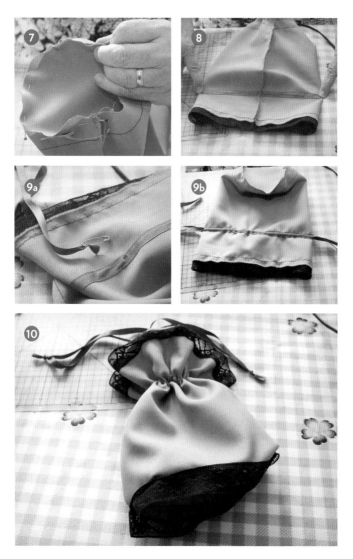

can sew a zigzag stitch onto them. Otherwise, just trim off any loose threads.

7) It is now time for the trickiest part of the process: connecting the bottom of the bag to the body. Before stitching, make sure the bag is inside out, then pin the two parts together, but make sure that the lace is pushed out of the way; otherwise it will be caught into the stitching, and you'll have to start again. Then when you stitch, do so approximately 1/2 inch from the edge.

8) Turn the bag the right side out, in order to make sure everything is neat and the lace is not trapped into the stitching. Then turn inside out again, and lay the bag on the table, fabric flat and the seam upward.

9a) You now need to make four slits in the bias binding: one on either side of the seam (to allow the ribbon to pass over),

one on the left of the bag, and one on the right. Then cut the ribbon in half, and attach a small safety pin to the end of one of the pieces.

9b) Thread it through one of the side holes, and follow it around until it comes back out of the original hole. Then do the same with the other ribbon, this time going in through the other side hole.

10) Tie the ends of the ribbons together, to create handles. Then turn the bag the right side out, and pull the ribbons outward to gather the top of the bag together.

You now have your own Marilyn-inspired drawstring bag.

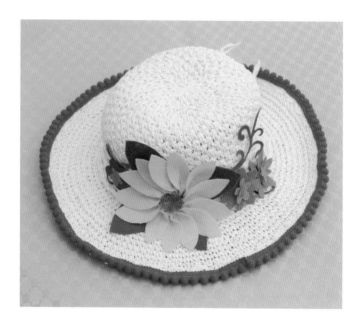

DECORATE A HAT

While tending to her garden at Fifth Helena Drive, Marilyn loved to wear a Mexican hat, complete with a bold flower decoration. Here is how you can decorate your own hat, in a Marilyn-inspired way.

WHAT YOU WILL NEED:

- ○ straw hat
- ○ felt in assorted colors
- ○ cardboard
- ○ pen

- ○ scissors
- ○ glue gun or needle and thread
- ○ colorful braid (optional)

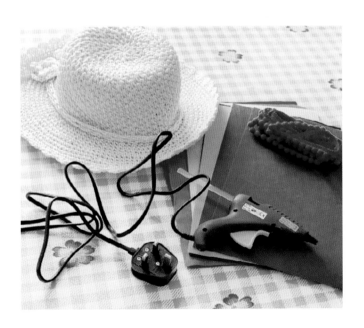

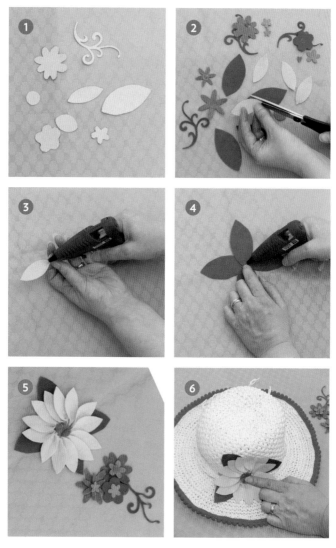

1) Draw petals, stems, and small flowers onto a piece of cardboard, and cut them out to make templates. You can be as creative as you like, so don't feel obliged to stick to our designs.

2) Carefully draw the shapes onto your felt, and cut them out. We made thirteen large petals, four green leaves, and a center circle for each large flower, then cut out a variety of stems and other smaller decorations.

3) Take each flower petal and fold it in half. Then glue or stitch at one end, so that it creates a 3-D effect.

4) Take your four leaves, and glue or stitch them together at the center and then start applying your petals. Make sure your petals touch in the middle, so that it is easy to glue or stitch on your center dot once all of the petals are in place.

5) Once you have created as many flowers as you need, simply glue or stitch them onto the hat.

6) We also stitched a braid around the edge, to give it added color. Your Marilyn-inspired hat is now ready to wear!

FOUR

beauty

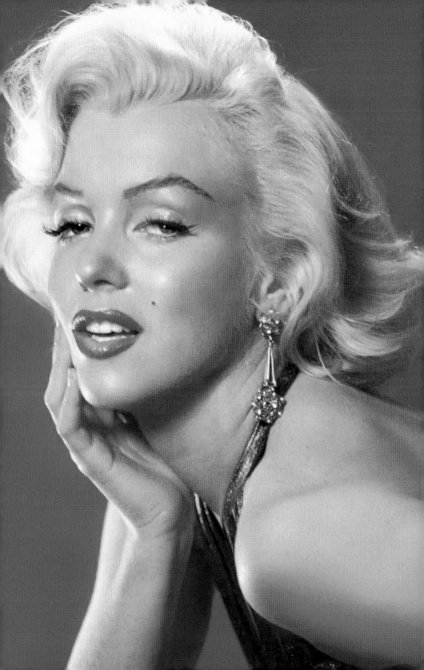

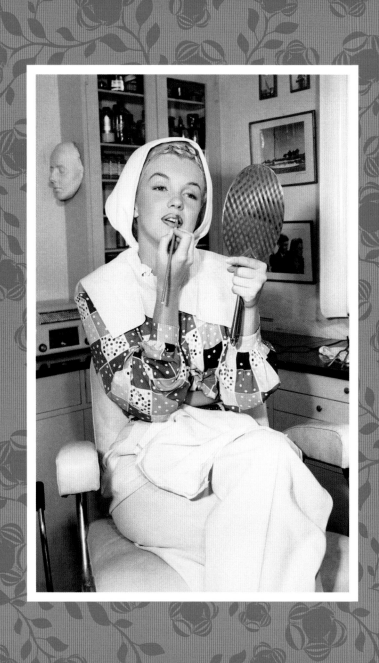

For Marilyn, wearing makeup was not as important as one may think. Her everyday appearance was often no more than a layer of cream or a touch of mascara. However, when she did dress up, Marilyn could spend hours perfecting her makeup, often with many different shades of lipstick, false eyelashes, and an array of eyeshadows. Many items from her makeup case have been sold at auction in the years since her death, revealing Marilyn's favorite colors and brands.

For eyes, the actress enjoyed Elizabeth Arden's cream eyeshadows—Autumn Smoke and Pearly Blue were among her favorites. Then there were eyeliners from the same manufacturer, in shades of brown and black. Stage makeup manufacturer Leichner of London provided light green eyeshadow, while nail polish came from Revlon in shades of Cherries à la Mode and Hot Coral. Marilyn liked Max Factor lipstick, cream makeup and cover-up from Anita d'Foged in a Day Dew shade, and perfumed lotion from the Quintess line by Shiseido.

For those wishing to wear the same brands as their idol, there are a number of options. The Quintess line is no longer available, but Shiseido still offers a large selection of creams and lotions. Elizabeth Arden doesn't make Autumn Smoke and Pearly Blue shadows anymore, but they do have a trio called Something Blue and another named Bronzed to

Be, which are similar in shade to the ones Marilyn wore. One Perfect Coral would be an appropriate Revlon alternative to Hot Coral, while Cherries in the Snow would replace Cherries à la Mode.

While many of the lines Marilyn chose are no longer manufactured, she would have no doubt been overjoyed that Max Factor recently created a range of lipsticks in her honor. Coming in four different shades—Marilyn Cabernet Red, Marilyn Ruby Red, Marilyn Sunset Red, and Marilyn Berry Red—the line gives fans the opportunity to find their own perfect color or combine several, just as the star herself did during the 1950s.

Marilyn used many different skin products, but perhaps her favorites were produced by Erno Laszlo. Marilyn returned time and time again to Laszlo and bought a vari-

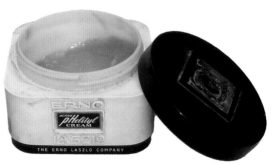

Marilyn's favorite skin products were from Erno Laszlo.

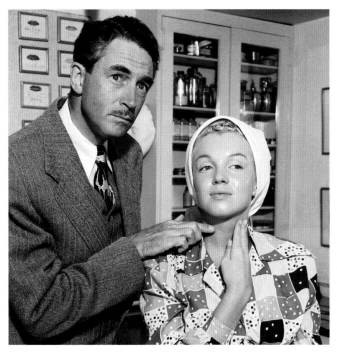

Healthy skin—important for any Hollywood star.

ety of his creations, which in the 1950s were available by
consultation only. During the 2005 auction of her posses-
sions at Julien's, a great many jars of Active Phelityl cream
were sold. Still available in remarkably similar packaging,
the Active Phelityl cream is one of Laszlo's original products and is a twenty-four-hour all-purpose product with
a pH value close to that of one's skin. The Laszlo website

109

celebrates famous clients such as Marilyn, Audrey Hepburn, and Jackie Kennedy, and it reveals that another of Marilyn's favorites was the Phormula 3-9 collection. The company now sells a box set featuring some of these products, along with artwork inspired by their iconic blonde client.

Collector Scott Fortner is fortunate enough to own some of Marilyn's Erno Laszlo cream. "There are still trails in the product from Marilyn's fingers," he says. "I call it my 'Marilyn was here' moment."

Marilyn was well-known for wearing Chanel No. 5 perfume, and photos of her holding the famous bottle are classics. However, there was another fragrance the private woman enjoyed just as much: Rose Geranium by London perfumer Floris. "Rose Geranium was introduced to the range in 1890, when pink geranium, palmarosa, and rose were added to the existing geranium scent," says Floris director Edward Bodenham.

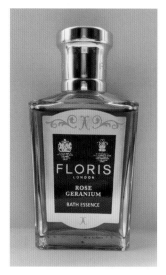

Marilyn discovered Floris perfume during her trip to England in 1956.

Marilyn discovered the perfume during her 1956 trip to London and instantly fell in love—so much so in fact that she continued to order it after she returned to the States. In 1959 she had six bottles shipped in just one order. The perfume was discontinued for a long time, though customers could still smell it in the form of bath essence. In 2017, however, it was returned as a hand-poured eau de toilette, available exclusively in the Jermyn Street store in London. "We are very touched that Marilyn visited the shop during her visit to England," says Edward, "and my grandfather was fortunate enough to have actually met her. We do occasionally have fans visiting the shop, especially to smell our Rose Geranium scent."

When one thinks of the iconic Marilyn hairdo, we generally picture the 1952–1953 look of *Gentlemen Prefer Blondes* and *How to Marry a Millionaire*. This was all about large waves just above the shoulder, with the top of the hair flicked over to the right. If you were to order a Marilyn wig from a costume retailer, it is likely that this is what you would receive. However, as with most women, Marilyn's hair changed significantly over the years. Here are just some of her looks:

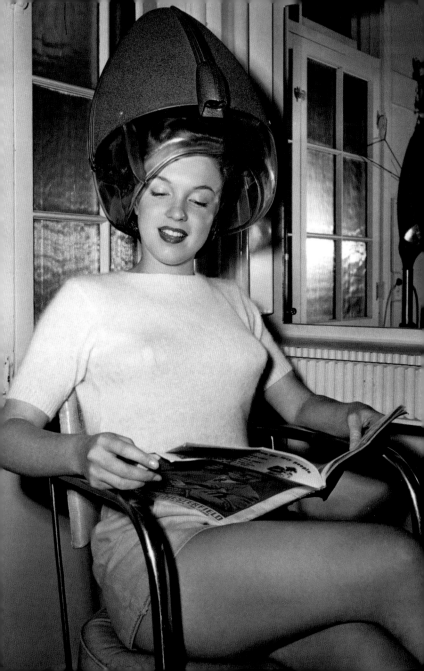

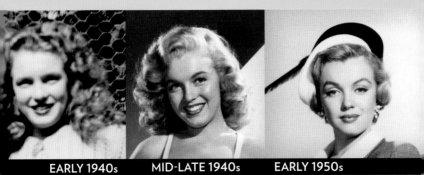

EARLY 1940s   **MID-LATE 1940s**   **EARLY 1950s**

Long brunette curls worn at or just below the shoulder. The hair was mainly left down, but occasionally would be braided or include a bow on the top of the head.

The Monroe hair really took shape during this time. It was short, golden blonde, and often worn in a sleek or wavy bob.

Various shades of blonde, with the curls relaxed into waves and worn below the shoulders. Marilyn would sometimes wear a scarf tied at the nape of the neck or pull her hair into a ponytail with a colorful bow.

OPPOSITE: It is safe to say that Marilyn spent many hours under the dryer to perfect her look.

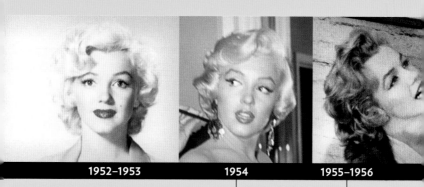

1952–1953   **1954**   **1955–1956**

The aforementioned signature Marilyn hairdo.

In The Seven Year Itch, *Marilyn's hair was seen in several different ways, from a sleek bob to messy platinum curls. When Madonna performed on her* Blond Ambition *tour thirty-five years later, the curls she sported in the latter half of the tour were reminiscent of Marilyn's in that film.*

This was the height of Marilyn's rebellion against Hollywood and the studio system, and it showed in her hair. Often looking as though she had just stumbled out of bed, her hair was pillowcase blonde, with large curls worn layered and just above the shoulders. In mid- to late 1956, while making Bus Stop *and* The Prince and the Showgirl, *her hair was shorter and in a strawberry-blonde shade.*

114

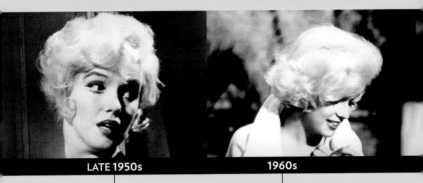

LATE 1950s   **1960s**

Marilyn embraced the 1960s with full gusto. One of her hairdressers, Kenneth Battelle, enjoyed giving her a white-blonde shade, blow-dried into side layers with lots of volume. However, the messy blonde at the heart of Marilyn's personality would sometimes rebel against the structured design, and she would instead wear her hair softly brushed out.

Marilyn's look during this era was one of grace and beauty, and that was often reflected in a more relaxed style. However, her longer hair was tied back into a French roll for much of the movie Some Like It Hot, *which depicted her as a singer in a 1920s girl band.*

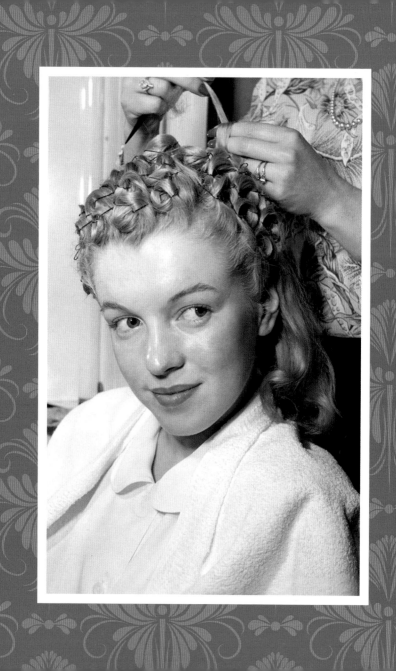

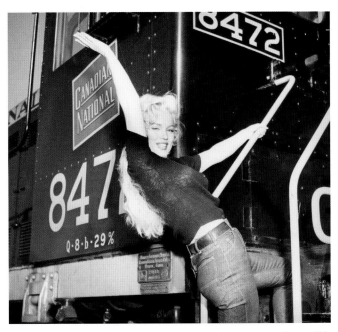

Her long hair was one of the very few things Marilyn liked about *River of No Return*. OPPOSITE: Pin-curling was a popular way of styling hair in the 1950s.

Once she achieved stardom, Marilyn became something of a poster girl for shorter hairstyles. However, occasionally film roles required longer locks, and in her role as Kay in *River of No Return* she sported the lengthiest style of her career. When asked where the long hair had come from, Marilyn replied, "Makeup department, of course. They put it on for me, every day, because I have to wear my hair with a bun in the back and there's not enough of it. Now I like it long, so at the end of the day I just let it down and parade around as it if were my own. When I get some time off between pictures, I'm going to sit around and grow my own."

Marilyn devotee Rebecca Swift has played with many different looks. "Over the years, I've done pretty much everything! For many, many years I was blonde and did 'Marilyn hair' every day. Now I'm a little older, I'm no longer blonde, but still influenced by Marilyn, and vintage or retro-styling in general." It isn't just the hair or even the outfits that interest Rebecca, however. "I also have a massive passion for jewelry, handbags, and shoes, whether true vintage or vintage style, and of course I love doing vintage makeup. A cat-eye flick and red lipstick always make your confidence soar."

Marilyn's body shape has always been a topic of discussion. In the 1990s it was claimed that she was the equivalent of a US size 16 in today's measurements, but this is simply untrue. The first document we have to show Marilyn's size comes from a 1945 entry in the Blue Book Agency records. According to agency boss Emmeline Snively, nineteen-year-old Norma Jeane's measurements were 36"-24"-34" and she weighed 120 pounds. In 1954, Marilyn's ID card listed her as 118 pounds, and while there is no documentary evidence as to her weight in the late 1950s, photographs show that Marilyn was slightly heavier at that time. However, by 1962, she was back to 117 pounds.

Marilyn expert Scott Fortner has taken measurements of the Marilyn garments he owns in order to determine her

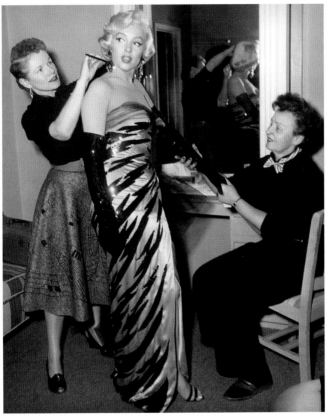

Marilyn has her hair done on the set of *The Seven Year Itch*.

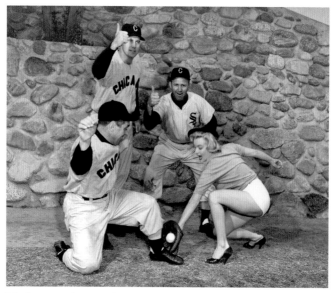

Marilyn was photographed with baseball players on several occasions. In fact it was a baseball-themed picture that first attracted the attention of Joe DiMaggio.

true size. Scott's investigation shows that in 1951, Marilyn's belt measured 27 inches when fastened. A skirt from 1953 was the same size, and a dress she wore in 1959 (one of her heaviest years), measured a still-tiny 28-1/2 inches.

For those wishing to eat like Marilyn, here are some of the meals she enjoyed during her lifetime: steak, lamb chops, liver, spaghetti, hamburgers, hot dogs, eggs, lobster, bagels, rye bread, grapefruit, and cheese sandwiches.

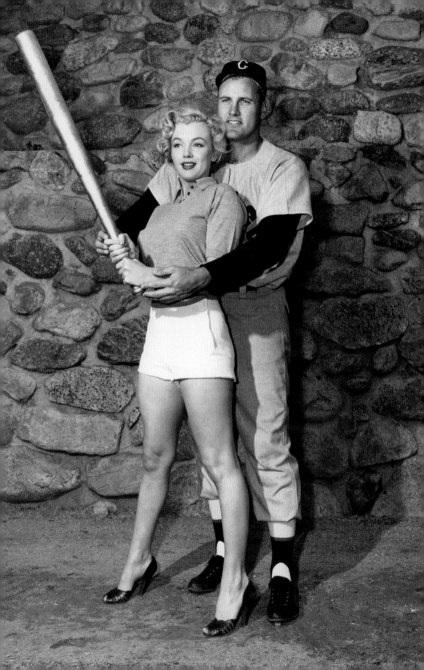

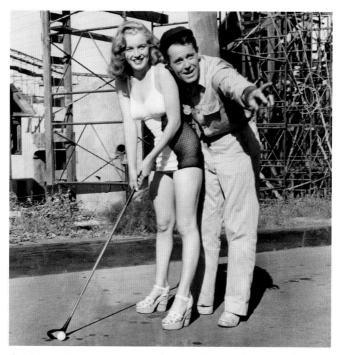

Celebrity golf events were a good way to be seen during her days as a young starlet.

Marilyn's favorite snack was caviar, but she didn't care much for olives or pastries, even though she offered them to guests. Favorite drink? Why, champagne of course, and Dom Pérignon in particular.

While we can't all have a figure like Marilyn's, we can take a leaf out of her book when it comes to exercise. From the beginning, she was a poster girl for fitness. As a teenager Norma Jeane was known to go horseback-riding, hiking, skiing, and swimming with her first husband, James Dougherty. Later she played golf with Joe DiMaggio and then enjoyed playing badminton with Arthur Miller's children and her friends Hedda and Norman Rosten.

Marilyn enjoyed playful sports but was not really interested in serious games. Exercise, however, was a big deal. "I am a great believer in exercise, just to 'keep things in proportion,'" she said in the early 1950s. "I am the lucky possessor of a small waist and some curves in the right places, but although I owe a lot to nature, I also owe a great deal to careful exercise, plenty of fresh fruit, and the right diet."

The "careful exercise" Marilyn spoke about involved weights, running, and yoga. More than thirty years before the world marveled at the sight of Jane Fonda's workout video or Madonna jogging through London's Hyde Park, Marilyn was photographed running around the back streets of Beverly Hills wearing jeans and a bikini top. Other photo shoots involved her tackling a variety of yoga positions (a rare practice in 1950s America) and lifting weights. The skeptical among us may wonder if it was all a publicity stunt, but an auction of Marilyn's belongings confirmed that she did actually own a workout bench and weights at the end of her life.

Marilyn often exercised in the privacy of her own home and also employed a yoga teacher by the name of Virginia Dennison. If you want to practice yourself, it is important to find a qualified instructor who will guide you through each asana in a safe manner. However, for those interested in knowing exactly what kind of positions Marilyn practiced, photographs from the time show her doing a shoulder stand, bow, plow, handstand, boat, forward bends, and twists.

Finally, to take away the aches and pains of a grueling workday, Marilyn had masseur Ralph Roberts, who would massage her privately and on the sets of movies. Marilyn often had trouble sleeping, so the therapy was designed not only to relieve muscles but to help her relax, too. Deeply dedicated to his employer, Ralph became Marilyn's trusted friend and spent many hours with her over the years. He later recalled shopping on Rodeo Drive with Marilyn, while she was in a disguise of comfortable slacks, blouse, and kerchief hiding her hair.

For those wishing to see Ralph Roberts on-screen, check out the scene in *The Misfits* in which Montgomery Clift's character is left concussed at the rodeo. Ralph plays an ambulance driver who cares briefly for the injured Montgomery.

OPPOSITE: Yoga was not yet a popular Western world pastime in the 1950s, but Marilyn practiced it.

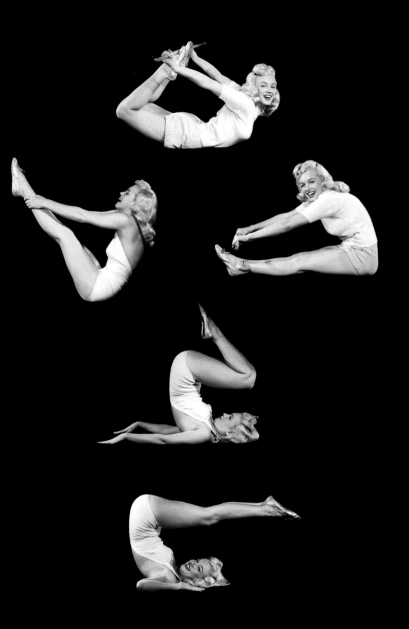

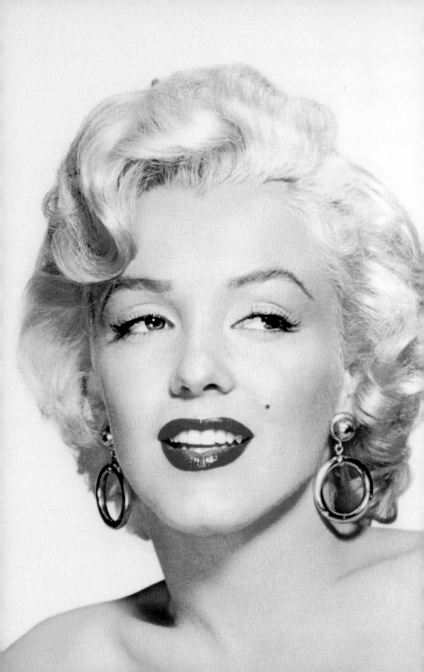

A MARILYN MAKEOVER:
the iconic look

SUZIE KENNEDY IS THE WORLD'S FOREMOST MARILYN Monroe tribute artist. She has worked extensively in television and film (most recently as Marilyn in *Blade Runner 2049*) and has worn the actress's outfits in both media and auction events. A fan and collector for many years, Suzie credits Marilyn as a huge inspiration and recognizes the positive influence the star has had on her life. Here Suzie re-creates Marilyn's most famous look, so that we can all put a bit of *Mmmm* into our makeup routine!

HAIR

WHAT YOU WILL NEED:

- a variety of large and medium curlers

- volume-boosting mousse

- thickening spray

- hair spray

- hair dryer

- soft brush

127

1a) After washing and lightly towel-drying your hair, apply volume-boosting mousse, and then put your hair into rows of curlers. You will need smaller curlers at the sides and back, larger ones on top and at the front.

1b) Marilyn wore her legendary layered wave to the right, so make sure you roll the curlers in that direction if you want an authentic style, or go with the flow of your own hair if it wants to go left.

2) Once curlers are in place, blow-dry for approximately twenty minutes, until hair is completely dry.

Tip: Once blow-drying is complete, you may want to do your makeup before removing the curlers. This will give a little extra time for the curls to take hold.

3a and b) Remove all of the curlers. If you want *The Seven Year Itch* hair, you might like to stop here. If not, keeping going.

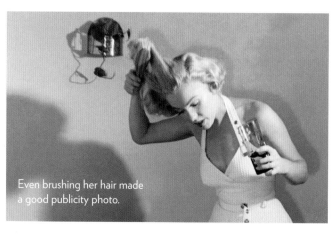

Even brushing her hair made a good publicity photo.

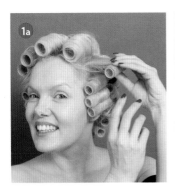

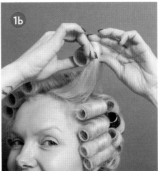

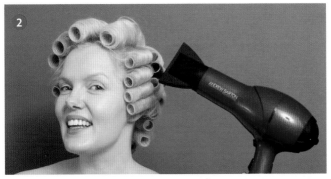

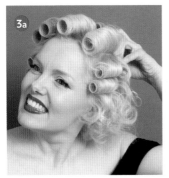

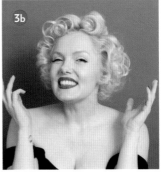

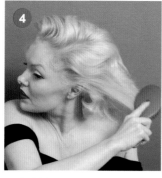

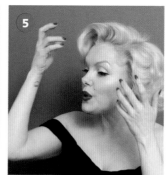

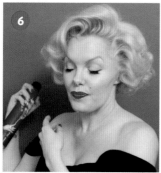

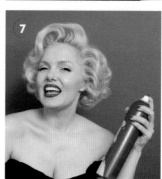

4) With a soft brush, sweep the hair down at the sides and then over at the top to create the famed Monroe flick.

5) Using your fingers, gently tease the hair until it is just right.

6) Apply a thickening spray over the entire head. This will create layers and make your hair more voluminous. Suzie uses Get Layered by Sexy Hair.

7) Finish with hair spray to hold.

OPPOSITE: In this early photo, Marilyn's hair is worn long.

130

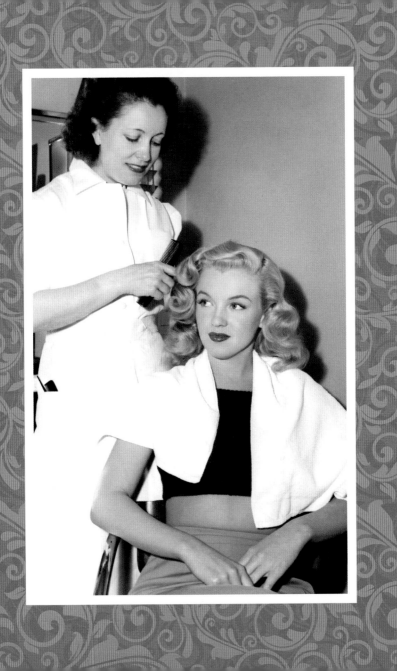

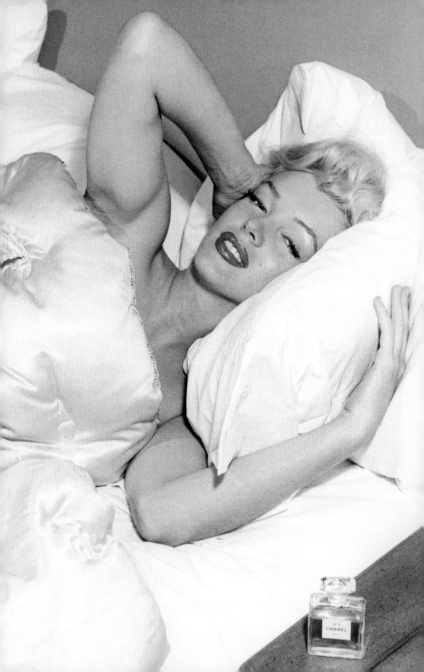

MAKEUP

WHAT YOU WILL NEED:

- ○ a good moisturizer
- ○ foundation
- ○ pressed powder
- ○ eyebrow pencil
- ○ concealer
- ○ highlighter
- ○ white eye shadow
- ○ liquid eyeliner
- ○ mascara

- ○ corner lashes and lash glue
- ○ natural-color blusher
- ○ soft burgundy lip pencil
- ○ dusty pink lip pencil
- ○ dark red lip pencil
- ○ medium red lipstick
- ○ nude/beige lipstick
- ○ nude lip gloss
- ○ toothpick

"In my view, most girls look more desirable with glistening lids and a moist mouth. A drop of oil on the lids will give the effect, and if you are handy with a lipstick brush, there's nothing like it for that luscious look."

—MARILYN

OPPOSITE: Marilyn's favorite perfumes were Rose Geranium by Floris and Chanel No 5.

1) First of all, make sure your skin is well-moisturized. Suzie does not wear a primer, but if that is part of your personal routine, apply that too.

2) Now it's time for foundation. Suzie uses M.A.C.'s Studio Fix shade NW10, which has a pink tint and gives a natural matte finish, but you'll want to pick a shade that suits your own skin tone. Using your applicator of choice (brush, sponge, or fingers, as Suzie uses), apply the product to the back of the hand first, and then tap it all over your face, until it appears flawless. Don't forget to blend it well into the neckline, to avoid any unsightly lines.

3) Once you're happy with the foundation, apply a liberal coat of pressed powder, using a sponge. Suzie's powder of choice is Chanel.

4) Eyebrows are next. Marilyn's brows had a natural point in the middle, which was distinctive. However, it is important to work with your own natural shape; otherwise it could go disastrously wrong. Some imitators color the brows black, but they should actually be brown, which of course matched Marilyn's natural hair color and looked good even as she went lighter blonde in the '50s. Using a brow pencil (Suzie likes to use M.A.C.), gently trace your eyebrows with delicate strokes, until they are filled in fully but not too harshly.

5) Apply a flesh-colored concealer to the eye lid, blending well with your finger. Then apply a small amount of highlighter just below the eyebrow to the brow bone and then onto the lid. This gives a luminous sheen to the upper eye, rather than the powdered appearance that comes from eyeshadow.

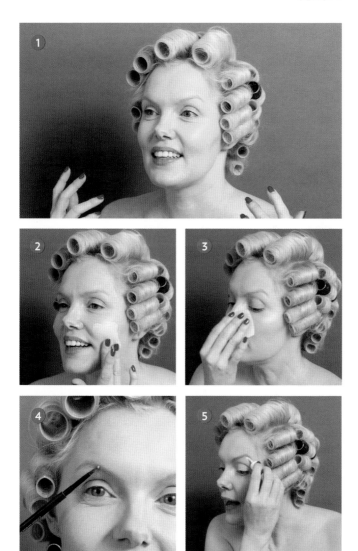

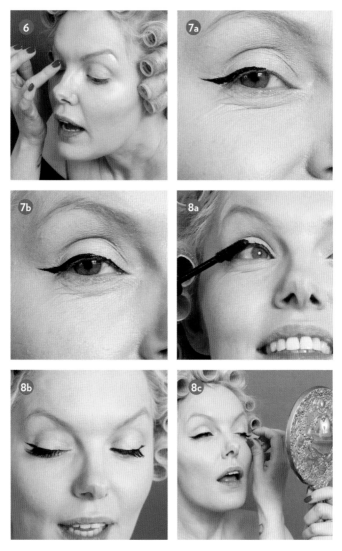

6) Apply a white eyeshadow (Suzie uses Boots No. 7) onto the lid of your eye. Here again Suzie prefers to use her finger rather than a brush, as she feels this gives her better coverage.

7a) Time for eyeliner. Marilyn's was more delicate than some of the other 1950s bombshells, so it's important to bear that in mind when applying. Using a black, liquid eyeliner, carefully draw a thin line outward from the middle of the eye, and add a small flick that extends past the eye itself.

7b) Then go back to the middle of the eye, and using a small "dotting" motion, apply more liner until you get a smooth and complete—but not thick—line. Tidy up any mistakes with a cotton swab. Repeat on the other eye.

8a) Give your lashes a coat of black mascara (Suzie uses Chanel), and then grab your false eyelashes. Tip: Suzie has studied Marilyn's makeup extensively and is sure that the actress herself used corner lashes, rather than a full set.

8b and c) Take the lashes, apply the correct lash glue, and then carefully stick them halfway along your eye, so that they reach the outer edge. This may take some practice, but persevere: the lashes really help finish your makeup. Don't put the glue away—you'll need it again in a moment!

9) Blush is next. Marilyn wore a natural shade, and Suzie likes to use a multicolored palette called Love At First Blush by Soap and Glory. Swish a brush around the product to gain a liberal amount of powder, then dust off the excess, and apply to the apples of the cheeks. Then travel upward toward the temples, all the time making sure that the blush is evenly blended.

10) Suzie's "Marilyn lips" are a work of art. So we'll take it slowly and in stages. First, carefully outline your lips with a soft burgundy–colored pencil. Suzie uses Half-Red from M.A.C.

11) Next take a dusty pink lip pencil (Suzie likes Lip Cheat Pillow Talk from Charlotte Tilbury), and completely fill the lip with color.

12) A dark red lip pencil is next. Suzie uses Brick from M.A.C., which is a golden red color. Carefully apply this inside the original lip liner, toward the edges of the lips.

13) Now for a medium red lipstick. Suzie uses Lady Bug from M.A.C. to fill the lips with color.

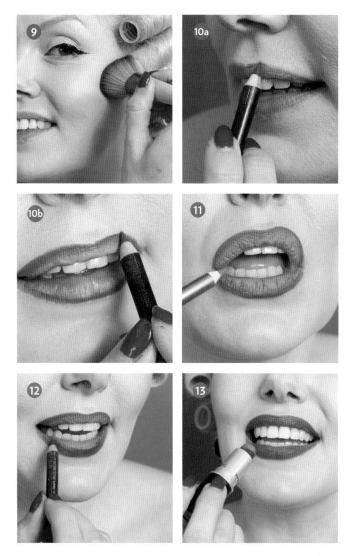

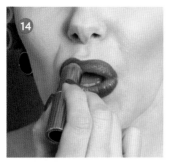

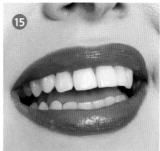

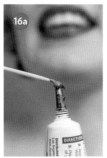

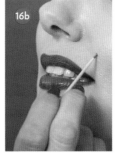

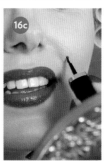

14) The last lipstick is a nude or beige shade. Charlotte Tilbury's Penelope Pink is the color Suzie goes for, which is described on the website as a "nude lipstick with pink undertones." You don't need a lot of this product. Simply dot a small amount onto the middle of the top and bottom lips, to give depth.

15) Finish the lips with a nude gloss. For Suzie, that means Seduction by Charlotte Tilbury. Using the applicator provided, run a layer of gloss over the lips to create a beautiful sheen.

16) One of the most famous of Marilyn's features is, of course, her beauty mark. This is where we need the eyelash glue again.

Squeeze a small amount of glue onto the end of your toothpick, then gently dab it onto your cheek to create an authentic-seeming bump. Marilyn's beauty mark was on her left side, between the mouth and nose, just on the edge of her cheek. Once the glue is set, take your liquid eyeliner and add a little color to the spot.

17) Now your iconic Marilyn look is complete except for one tiny detail—a spritz of Chanel No. 5 of course!

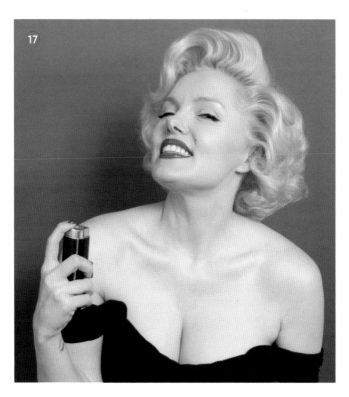

FIVE

life skills

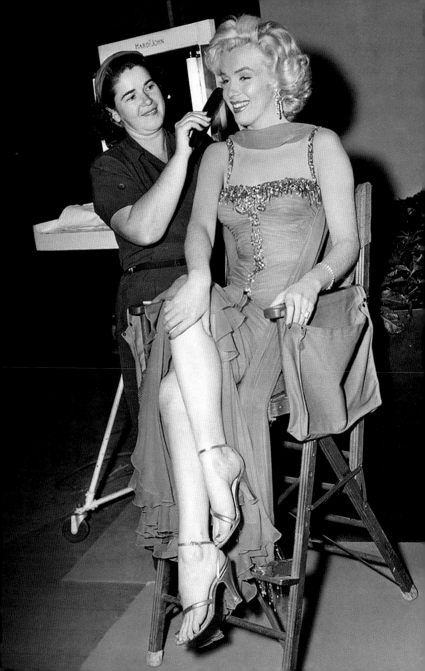

Some people make the mistake of seeing Marilyn as a victim of Hollywood, somebody who had little intellect and was easily taken advantage of. That is simply untrue. Although Marilyn did have a tragic end and endured unhappy times, she was actually a remarkably strong woman. She always strived to do her best; she was not afraid to speak her truth or stand up for what she believed in. We can learn many lessons from studying how Marilyn conducted herself in her public and private lives. Here are just some of them.

KNOWLEDGE IS POWER

Marilyn never finished high school, but that did not stop her from seeking out knowledge and education throughout her life. This thirst took many forms. In 1946, when newly signed to Twentieth Century Fox, Marilyn took courses that were provided by the studio for their fledgling actors. Many starlets skipped these classes in favor of hanging out at the beach or lying in bed late, but Marilyn soaked up everything offered to her. When she was asked why she went to class instead of relaxing, her answer was clear: if an opportunity to act came along, she needed to be ready.

After her Fox contract was terminated in 1947, the starlet eventually found herself at Columbia, where she met acting coach Natasha Lytess. Although the woman was stern and at times even possessive, Marilyn studied with her from 1948 until 1954. During these years, the young actress also took lessons at the Actors Lab, had private classes with teacher Michael Chekhov, and experimented with a few group workshops with actors such as Charles Laughton. The former she enjoyed immensely, but the latter she found a little intimidating and did not become a regular guest.

"It is the biggest waste of anyone's time to keep looking back. To think about what is happening right now, and what is coming up in the future, is much healthier." —MARILYN

The Bliss-Hayden Miniature Theatre became an important part of Marilyn's life in the late 1940s. Determined to gain as much acting experience as she could, she was a regular attendee and was cast in at least two plays: the first was *Glamour Preferred*, which ran from October 12 to November 2, 1947, and the second was *Stage Door*, performed in the summer of the following year.

In 1951, Marilyn attended art appreciation and literature courses at the University of California, Los Angeles. Her teacher for the latter was Claire Soule, and the course took place Thursday evenings from seven to nine p.m. Marilyn enjoyed the classes, but it wasn't long before fellow students recognized her and began gazing at the actress more than the teacher. When they became too inquisitive, she decided to quit, though she always intended to return one day. She even enrolled in a mail-in art class during the late 1950s.

While she was always searching for knowledge, perhaps the most famous of her alliances came when Marilyn attended the Actors Studio in New York. The actress was keen to explore different ways of acting, and she dreamt of one day appearing in a Broadway play. Sadly for us all, that was one goal she did not fulfill, but Marilyn's association with Lee Strasberg, his wife, Paula, and the other actors at the studio has become legendary. In fact, when the actress appeared in a scene from Eugene O'Neill's play *Anna Christie*, it was so successful that fellow students could hardly believe that such talent and emotion had come from the quiet woman who liked to sit in the back and take notes.

WHEN IN DOUBT, READ A BOOK

While many of Marilyn's film roles were of a dumb-blonde nature, the woman herself was anything but. A lover of classic literature, she had an enormous book collection that included heavyweight authors such as William Shakespeare, Leo Tolstoy, James Joyce, and Anton Chekhov. Famous photographs taken in the 1950s show Marilyn reading in a variety of places, including a park, a university library, her home, and a bookshop. "I read most every chance I get," she said.

Marilyn's notes, thoughts, poems, and artwork were published in several works: *Fragments* (2010) and *Girl Waiting* (2012). Since we only otherwise have a ghost-written autobiography (*My Story*, written in 1954), *Fragments* and *Girl Waiting* offer a spectacular glimpse into the real-life person. This has proved immensely important in a world where Marilyn Monroe is often unfairly dismissed as a dim-witted blonde with no substance.

In the books, which are based on a series of journals found in Marilyn's belongings after her death, readers can discover her notes on life, work, relationships, and interests. Her intellectual side is revealed in book suggestions, her homebody personality shines through in shopping lists and recipes, and her caring nature is everywhere present in notes reminding her to buy birthday presents or send greetings to friends. Marilyn's notebooks show a woman of great depth and intelligence, a human being intent on finding her place in the world and achieving greatness in acting and life.

To get a sense of just how intelligent and interested in the world Marilyn was, one need only take a look at her collection of books, many of which have been sold at auction. Here are just some of the volumes Marilyn acquired during her lifetime:

Man's Supreme Inheritance by F. Matthias Alexander
The Fall by Albert Camus
Camille by Alexandre Dumas
The Great Gatsby by F. Scott Fitzgerald
Ulysses by James Joyce *(Marilyn was photographed by Eve Arnold while reading this book)*
The Prophet by Kahlil Gibran
Man Against Himself by Karl A. Menninger
Sons and Lovers by D. H. Lawrence
Death in Venice and Seven Other Stories by Thomas Mann
A Farewell to Arms by Ernest Hemingway
The Short Reign of Pippin IV by John Steinbeck
The Philosophy of Plato

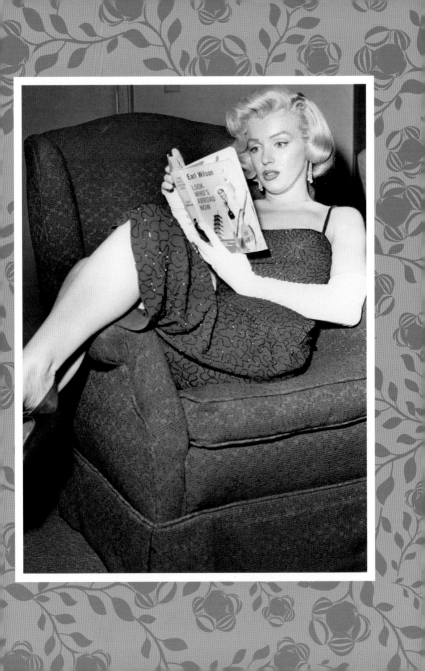

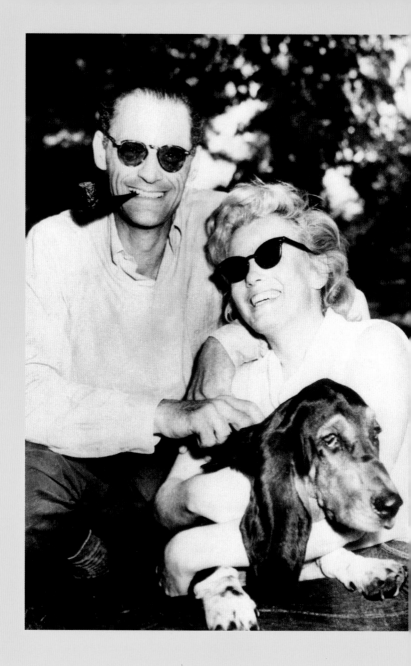

BE KIND TO ANIMALS AND CHILDREN

Because of her upbringing—which the actress often described as being deprived of kisses and hugs—Marilyn had a great empathy for children and animals. Over the course of her life, the actress had a variety of pets, including a basset hound called Hugo, a parakeet named Butch, and a Maltese pup called Maf. However, her love for furry and feathered friends went much deeper than owning pets. Over the years, many people have come forward to describe how she saved the lives of animals in need. These excursions included chasing a hawk that was terrorizing a neighborhood swallow and her babies, throwing stranded fish back into the water while walking on the beach, and trying to buy a calf from a farmer who intended to sell it for meat. When her efforts with the cow failed, Marilyn became absolutely distraught.

Her love for children ran just as deep. The actress had three stepchildren—Joe DiMaggio Jr. with second husband Joe, and Jane and Bobby Miller with third husband Arthur. During the DiMaggio marriage, Marilyn would often take the young Joe to the swimming pool, and then during the

OPPOSITE: Hugo was Marilyn's beloved basset hound. She worried frequently about his mental health.

151

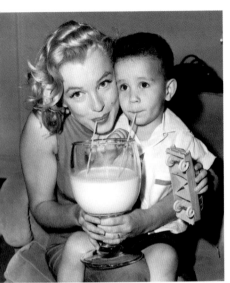 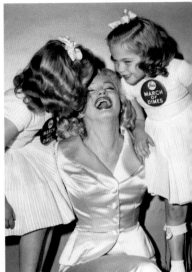

Miller marriage, she entertained her stepchildren with letters written in the voice of the family dog, Hugo.

Even after she had divorced their fathers, Marilyn kept
in regular contact with the children. She discussed politics
with Bobby Miller and even spoke to Joe Jr. on the night
of her death. The young man called to tell her that he had
recently broken off a relationship with his girlfriend, a
woman Marilyn apparently didn't care for.

Her stepchildren weren't the only kids in Marilyn's
life. Over the years she made friends with various others,
including the children of friends such as photographer

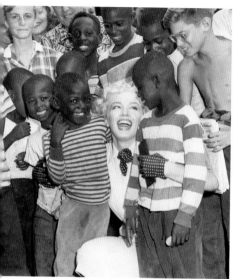 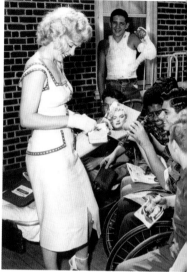

FROM FAR LEFT: In 1957, Marilyn took part in a charity event for the Milk Fund. • In 1958, Marilyn attended the annual March of Dimes fashion show. • Some happy children meet Marilyn in Atlantic City. • Marilyn signs autographs at the Betty Bacharach Home for Afflicted Children in 1952.

Sam Shaw and poet Norman Rosten. Her charity work often revolved around organizations associated with children and orphanages (including the one she lived in as a child, Hollygrove); WAIF, an organization that found adoptive parents for abandoned children; the Milk Fund for Babies; and a benefit at the Hollywood Bowl organized to raise money for underprivileged children.

ALWAYS TAKE THE HIGH ROAD

Marilyn famously said that it was the people who made her a star, but some were not too happy about her success. Actress Joan Crawford was a big detractor and poured scorn over everything from an outfit worn at an award ceremony to her general demeanor. Even though the words were hurtful, Marilyn never lowered herself to Crawford's level. Instead, she expressed her sadness to journalist Louella Parsons, who printed her thoughts; Marilyn immediately gained public sympathy.

While she often seethed about costars and directors in private, in public she would always remain respectful. During the making of *The Prince and the Showgirl* with Laurence Olivier, the two were often seen quarrelling, and Marilyn stormed off the set on at least one occasion. However, the actress saw this as a private affair, and when she left London in November 1956, she declared the work a magnificent success, kissed the actor on the cheek, and left without any stern words toward her nemesis.

DON'T BE A DOORMAT

While Marilyn was publicly gracious to those she did not care for, that did not mean she was weak or unable to speak for herself. Far from it, in fact! Her first husband, James Dougherty, objected to his wife's modeling career and told her that the moment the war ended, they would settle down and have a family. She responded to this demand by heading to Las Vegas and filing for divorce before he returned. This was similar to her situation with base-ball star Joe DiMaggio. He knew when they first started dating that his girlfriend was a famous movie star, and it certainly did not stop him from marrying her. However, Joe's distaste for her movie career, and the control he tried to exert over the clothes she wore and the friends she had, did not sit well with Marilyn. When it all became too much, she divorced DiMaggio and, despite claims to the contrary, always said that she would never marry him again. Third husband Arthur Miller was a huge support to Marilyn when it came to her career, and for a time they lived happily together in New York and Connecticut. However, when he used her life experiences and personality as inspiration for the movie *The Misfits*, the fallout contributed to the breakdown of the marriage.

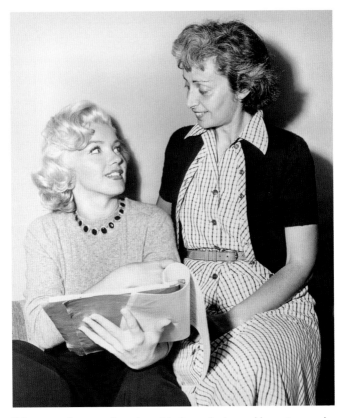

When something wasn't working, Marilyn walked away. Her acting coach Natasha Lytess was fired in 1954, when the actress moved to New York.

Marilyn's strength was also demonstrated in the way she dealt with her home studio, Twentieth Century Fox. During the making of *Gentlemen Prefer Blondes*, the (already famous) actress was not given a dressing room. Instead of just accepting the fact, Marilyn quite rightly complained bitterly until she was presented with one. Two years later she walked out on her contract when it was clear that Fox was anxious to typecast her, and later in her career, she spoke publicly about the studio's treatment of her and other actors. According to Marilyn, Fox treated actors as machines instead of human beings. This was something that made the actress furious.

Even business partner Milton Greene received the brunt of Marilyn's anger, when she questioned his motives within her company. The photographer was fired from his position on the board, and while she was always respectful when talking publicly about Greene, she did make clear that their partnership was not, in her opinion, working out.

The "don't be a doormat" philosophy was extended to the treatment of others, too. When Laurence Olivier openly criticized the performance of Susan Strasberg in the play *The Diary of Anne Frank*, Marilyn was the first to jump in and protect her friend. Then during the 1956 making of *The Prince and the Showgirl* in London, she overheard her security guard, P. C. Hunt, shouting at a young man hired to play piano at her home. Marilyn immediately told the guard that his behavior was out of order and privately apologized to her pianist.

TREASURE YOUR FRIENDS

Marilyn desperately wanted to be an actress, but once she achieved worldwide fame, she realized that it was not something that could sustain happiness for a lifetime. With that in mind, Marilyn treasured her relationships with friends like poet Norman Rosten and his wife, Hedda; teachers Lee and Paula Strasberg; photographer Sam Shaw; and even Joe DiMaggio (as a confidante, not as her husband). One of her greatest pleasures was spending time with friends while off duty, by picnicking on the beach, playing outdoor games, entertaining in her home, and talking about poetry, literature, and art.

Perhaps one of Marilyn's most enduring friendships was with her father-in-law, Isidore Miller. Having never known her real father, Marilyn would revel in taking care of "Dad," which included cooking his favorite dishes, inviting him to stay at her home, and writing him long, loving letters. Even after her divorce from Arthur Miller, Marilyn still called Isidore Dad and worried about his welfare after the death of his wife. One of her last vacations was when she met the older man for a break in Florida, and he was her companion on the evening she sang "Happy Birthday" to President John F. Kennedy. After Marilyn died, Isidore was shocked and bereaved, and a year later he spoke lov-

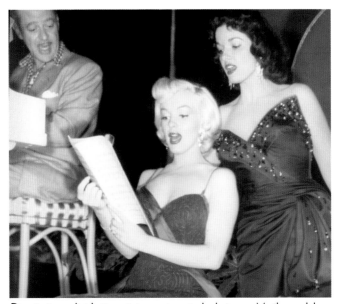

Despite journalists' attempts to create a rivalry between Marilyn and Jane Russell, they actually became good friends.

ingly about his surrogate daughter in an article published in *Good Housekeeping*.

Marilyn was also generous to her friends. If someone was in need of financial support, she would be the one to provide it. An example of this came when friend Norman Rosten needed investors for a play he'd written called *Mister Johnson*. Marilyn gave him the money and remained close friends with Rosten, even though the play folded after a matter of weeks. She was also generous with gifts.

159

Her notebooks show various reminders for birthdays and anniversaries. Similarly, if a friend took an interest in one of her belongings, Marilyn would either hand it over or buy another and send it as a gift.

In the mid-late 1950s, Arthur Miller felt the full extent of Marilyn's generosity when she stood by him when he faced contempt of Congress for not naming names during the McCarthy witch hunt against suspected Communists in the entertainment industry. Marilyn was warned that she could lose her career for standing beside Miller during the proceedings, but she refused to step away. As far as she was concerned, Arthur Miller needed her help and support, and she was more than happy to give it to him.

DON'T BE SCARED OF THE KITCHEN

It is fair to say that during her first marriage as a teenager to James Dougherty, Marilyn (or Norma Jeane, as she was still known then) was not the best of cooks. According to Dougherty, she would cook him peas and carrots every day, purely because she enjoyed the colors. This may have been

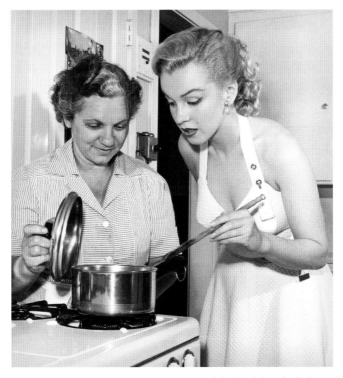

Although she was not a natural in the kitchen, Marilyn did gradually learn to cook.

an exaggeration on his part, but the fact remains that at the beginning of her adult life, Marilyn was not a big fan of the kitchen. But the actress persevered over the years, and by the time she met Joe DiMaggio, she had learned how to cook several Italian dishes, though this didn't always go to plan.

According to Marilyn herself, she once tried to make pasta noodles from scratch by following a recipe. Unfortunately, the text did not say how long to dry the noodles, and by the time her guests arrived, they were still soft and wet. Marilyn got out her hairdryer in an attempt to dry the food quickly, but instead sent the noodles flying all over the kitchen counter. She then had to scoop them all up and attempted to try again.

By the time Marilyn was married to Arthur Miller, she had become quite an expert in the kitchen and frequently cooked for his parents and friends. When asked by journalists why he had suddenly put on some weight, the playwright smiled and told them that it was because of general contentment and Marilyn's cooking. During this time, the actress added several cookbooks to her collection, most notably *The Joy of Cooking* by Irma S. Rombauer and a volume by Fannie Farmer. She would make breakfast every morning, and her notebook reveals an undated but planned dinner of beef, turkey, green salad, vegetables, potatoes, celery hearts, and radishes. Hors d'oeuvres would be caviar, and dessert consisted of fruit and ice cream.

A rather elaborate Thanksgiving stuffing recipe consisted of a mix of sourdough bread, meat, herbs, and nuts. Discovered long after her death, this recipe has since become a fan favorite; many try to reproduce it during the holiday season.

SOMETIMES LESS IS MORE

Although Marilyn was married three times during the course of her life, anyone who thinks she went in for huge Hollywood weddings full of glitz and sparkle would be wrong. Her marriage to James Dougherty took place on June 19, 1942, in the home of a family friend. The bride wore a long veil, a white, floor-length lace gown with long sleeves, full skirt, and ruffled neckline; she carried a bouquet of white gardenias. Norma Jeane loved the venue because there was a sweeping staircase from which she could descend, and she was given away by her foster mother, Aunt Ana.

Her marriage to Joe DiMaggio was even less pretentious. On January 14, 1954, Marilyn and Joe arrived at San Francisco City Hall with several witnesses and were married in just a few minutes by Judge Charles S. Peery. Outside, hundreds of fans waited for the couple to emerge and witnessed Marilyn run to Joe's Cadillac, wearing an unpretentious dark brown pencil suit with white ermine collar and a brooch at the neck. The bride also carried a small bouquet of orchids. The wedding preparations were not in any way elaborate, and in fact the

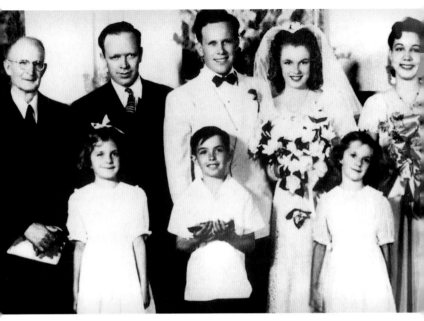

Norma Jeane married James Dougherty in a simple ceremony.

couple had only decided to get married some weeks earlier. The bride wore an outfit she had worn previously.

For her marriage to Arthur Miller, Marilyn had two ceremonies. The first was a humble affair and took place on the evening of June 29, 1956, at a White Plains, New York, courthouse. The bride wore probably the most modest of all her wedding outfits: a pink sweater and black skirt. Two days later, events were a bit more glamorous when Mr. and Mrs.

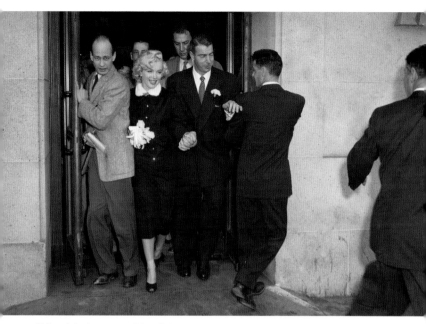

When Marilyn married Joe DiMaggio, her "something old" was her outfit.

Miller headed to the home of Arthur's agent, Kay Brown. There they were married in a Jewish ceremony followed by a beautiful garden party celebration, surrounded by friends and family. Footage of the event shows that Marilyn wore a white fitted gown with a low neckline, a short veil, and for at least some of the time, small, white gloves. The bride seemed to have great fun with the veil and was seen lifting and lowering it throughout the reception.

DON'T BE DRAWN INTO GOSSIP

One of the positive attributes that model agency boss Emmeline Snively noticed about Norma Jeane was her lack of interest in gossip. While some of the other models would gather in corners and partake in endless chatter, Norma Jeane would rather concentrate on her work and stay out of anything that would hurt or shame other people. This personality trait continued throughout her life, and while the press would often entice her into ranting about other female stars, they were left disappointed.

Two women pitted against Marilyn in the media were so-called rivals Diana Dors and Elizabeth Taylor. The press even went so far as to mention Dors during a press conference to announce Marilyn's marriage to Arthur Miller, but the actress assured them that she had never met Dors so was unqualified to comment.

Another sneaky effort to obtain gossip came when Marilyn was leaving a New York hospital in 1961, after suffering from emotional exhaustion. As reporters crowded around her, one unprofessional cad poked Marilyn with a newspaper featuring Elizabeth Taylor on the cover. Marilyn saw what he was doing and immediately whipped her arm (and

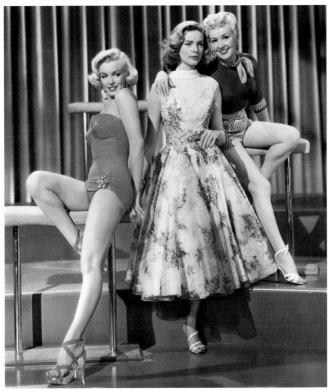

Marilyn, Lauren Bacall, and Betty Grable in *How to Marry a Millionaire*.

attention) away. Stalking film sets was a great way for the
press to try to stir up some tittle-tattle between actresses,
but once again Marilyn would never bite. In 1953, a rivalry
was attempted between Marilyn and her *How to Marry a
Millionaire* costars Lauren Bacall and Betty Grable. The

media efforts were unrewarded, however, and Marilyn even attended a party with Grable and the premiere of *Millionaire* with Bacall and her husband, Humphrey Bogart. Around the same time, reporters desperately wanted Marilyn and Jane Russell to fall out on the set of *Gentlemen Prefer Blondes*. Despite claims that the two women bitterly disliked each other, Marilyn and Jane became friends and always spoke highly of each other.

PUSH ON, EVEN WHEN YOU'RE SCARED

Marilyn is a glorious role model for pushing through, even in times of distress. The media made a great fuss about how Marilyn frequently arrived late on set and forgot her lines. However, while some would describe this as unprofessional, there is another way of looking at this behavior. Marilyn certainly wasn't the easiest actress to work with, but in spite of the fact that she was terrified of acting, she did it! She still showed up (eventually), still played the parts, and still studied relentlessly.

Many times Marilyn even worked at times of great heartache or pain. For instance, while making *Monkey Busi-*

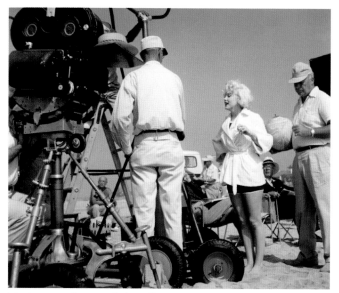

Marilyn was often terrified on film sets, but her final performance was always magical.

ness in 1952, she was suffering from appendicitis. Actor Bob Cornthwaite remembered director Howard Hawks insisting that Marilyn continue working. She did so, and her appendix was eventually removed after shooting had finished. A similar experience happened during *The Seven Year Itch*, when Marilyn was emotionally unwell after the collapse of her marriage to Joe DiMaggio. Once again she continued to work, and the performance she gave went down in history as one of her all-time best.

LOOK TO THE GREATS FOR INSPIRATION

Marilyn had many idols during her lifetime. These included Marlon Brando, Clark Gable, Charlie Chaplin, Greta Garbo, Ginger Rogers, Jean Harlow, Eleanora Duse, Carl Sandburg, Arthur Miller, Abraham Lincoln, Frank Sinatra, and Albert Einstein.

They say we should never meet our idols, but Marilyn was lucky enough to meet many of hers and actually become friends with some. Brando became a romantic interest, Gable was a costar in *The Misfits*, and Rogers worked with her in *Monkey Business*. Carl Sandburg became a close friend toward the end of Marilyn's life, and she even married Arthur Miller.

DREAM BIG

Raised in a series of foster homes and an orphanage, Marilyn did not have the most encouraging of starts. When she tentatively began her modeling career, she did so without the support of family and encountered much criticism for her hair color and style (too dark and curly), her nose (deemed too long), and her smile (so wide it revealed her

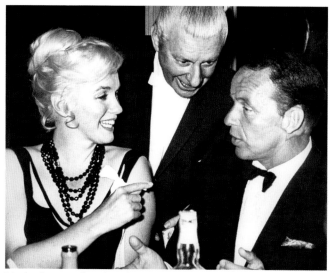
Marilyn became friends with several of her idols, including singer Frank Sinatra.

gums). These comments would be enough to send most people back to their day job, but Marilyn persevered.

The same can be said for when she eventually became famous. Forever told that she was only good enough to act in musicals and in dumb-blonde roles, Marilyn could have been forgiven for settling for those things. However, she had ambitions for much more, and despite threats and gossip from Twentieth Century Fox and the media, she moved to New York and set up her own film company. Not bad for a woman who grew up on the wrong side of the tracks!

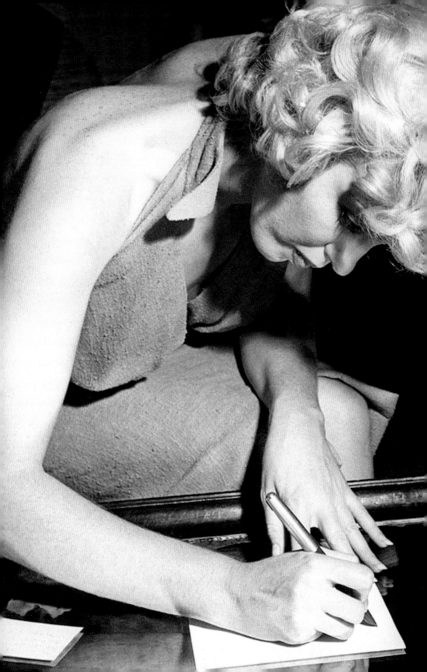

personal effects

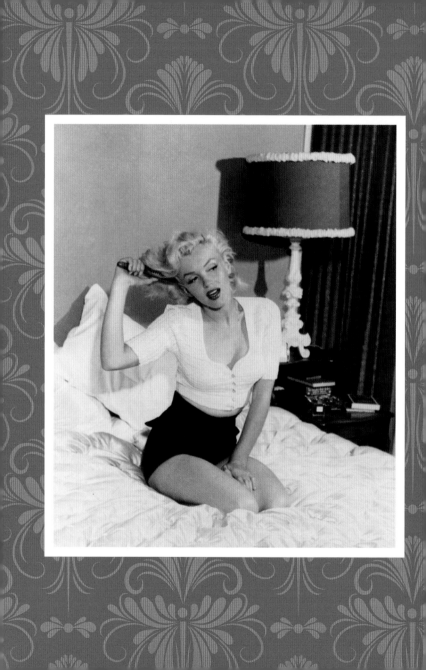

MARILYN AFICIONADOS ARE UNIQUE. WHILE many other fandoms like to emulate their idol's makeup or collect their photos and posters, we seem to go one stage further and enjoy collecting household items that either belonged to Marilyn or seem rather like something one would find in her home.

The actress's tastes were eclectic. In her Fifty-Seventh Street New York apartment there was a lot of glassware: ashtrays, vases, bowls, a candelabra, decanters, wine glasses, and even a glass toothpick holder. Also on display was a variety of works of art, including a gray stone torso on a marble base. A piano that had been bought by her mother in the 1930s stood handsomely as a centerpiece, and a deep, comfortable sofa played host to playwrights, producers, and poets. When her belongings were sold at auction in 1999, many regal items were among the lots, including beautiful chandeliers and a pair of Louis XV Provincial-style chairs.

"I like my home, and I am much more interested in it than people might suppose—yet that is natural, for having at last a place that is really my home is something I find very pleasant."—MARILYN

In her last home, at 12305 Fifth Helena Drive, Marilyn was in the process of decorating when she passed away. Pieces acquired for the house were mainly Mexican in origin, style, or both and included tapestry wall hangings, colorful wool throws, bright pottery and baskets, metal musician figures, colored glassware, and lots of chunky wooden furniture. Her February 1962 trip to Mexico proved beneficial for acquiring more beautiful items for her home, though much of the furniture would only arrive after Marilyn died.

Despite the many auctions dedicated to Marilyn's personal belongings, the steep prices and magnificent demand have led to most collectors being left out of these high-profile events. "I've never collected the personal items because I never had the means to," says Fraser Penny. "And I think it's great that people do that and exhibit them for everyone to see. It's a special field but it never occurred to me to do it, as whenever I saw them sell at auctions, it was for prices that I could never afford or would want to pay."

This is a dilemma for most would-be Marilyn collectors, and likely the reason look-alike items are so popular. I know some people who have bought extraordinary items, like nutcrackers or water tumblers and even tables and chairs, because they resemble Marilyn's. Several admirers pooled their funds to purchase a Mexican wall hanging purely because it was the same design as one Marilyn hung in her Fifth Helena Drive home.

Admirers often search for years for the one replica item they'd love to own. EBay is a great help in that regard, but with many aiming to buy the same piece, it can be a cutthroat and often disappointing business. What's great about collecting home furnishings rather than clothes is that there are still thousands of vintage items scattered all around the world that are similar in design to Marilyn's own belongings. Some older people tend to hold onto their ornaments until the end of their lives, and those that are not passed down through the generations end up being sold. Subscribing to auction house newsletters and scouring their catalogues whenever a new sale is imminent is exceptionally helpful when it comes to Marilyn-style collecting.

Marilyn's Mexican star light has become a must-have for fans.

Antiques and vintage fairs are another fantastic way of finding items similar to those Marilyn owned. I always take along photographs of Marilyn's belongings in the hope that I can find similar items, and I have been lucky on several occasions. It is also essential to scour local antique shops on a regular basis. My most precious find is a Mexican star lamp similar to one hanging in Marilyn's Fifth Helena Drive home, which I coveted for over thirty years.

The lamps are fairly easy to find in the United States—they have been spotted on Olvera Street in Los Angeles and in various household stores and websites. However, in England they are rare, and I had all but given up on ever finding one. Then one day my luck changed when I walked into a local antique shop. There in front of me was not one star lamp but two, and both had literally just arrived in store. I became so excited with my discovery that I told the shopkeeper all about their history. The woman then asked for a list of other Marilyn-related items I admire, and now keeps me up-to-date with any unique finds.

Using antique fairs and auctions is a highly effective way of finding vintage items that resemble Marilyn's. However, if you'd rather buy brand new articles, don't forget to check out your local home furnishing stores. Thanks to the persistent interest in mid-century designs, there are often modern-day

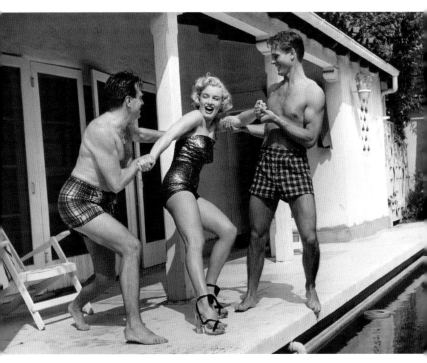

While several bathing suits have been sold at auction, the location of Marilyn's Lucite shoes remains a mystery.

replicas of popular housewares of the kind used by Marilyn, most commonly glassware, statues, and artwork.

Greg Schreiner, founder and president of the Marilyn Remembered fan club, was lucky to begin his collection before prices skyrocketed. "I started collecting Marilyn-owned items in 1984, when I attended my first

179

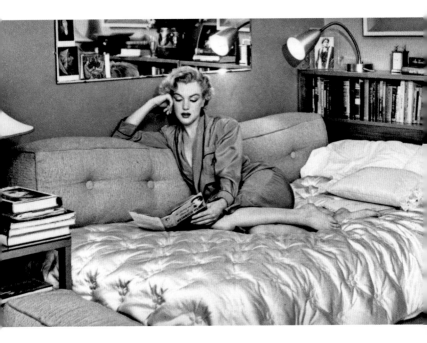

costume auction and acquired a red dress with purple sash that Marilyn wore to the premiere of *Monkey Business*. It was a thrilling moment and got me started seriously collecting real Marilyn items. I have many favorite pieces in my collection, and I love all of them. Asking to choose a favorite is somewhat like asking a mother who her favorite child is. I still continue to collect Marilyn, but her value has risen so much that I can no longer afford the big pieces I used to collect. Nevertheless, I still find an occasional piece that fits into my budget."

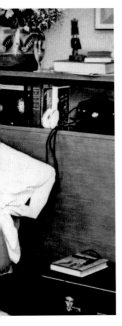
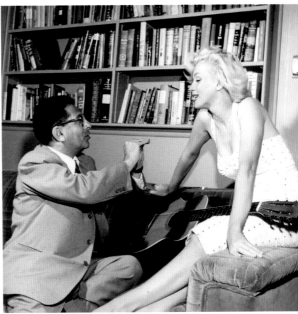

LEFT TO RIGHT: Marilyn is surrounded by her books and photos in this early photo. Marilyn had a huge book collection. She is seen here with reporter and friend Sidney Skolsky.

Marilyn enthusiast Vanessa Jayne Roden has been able to buy several items owned or related to her idol. "I purchased Marilyn's autograph almost three years ago now. I never thought in my wildest dreams I would get to own her autograph, as it can go for thousands and thousands at auction. I was overwhelmed with joy when I finally had it

181

in front of me (although it is quite faded), and I can quite proudly say I cried like a baby."

Even though Vanessa owns several authentic pieces, it still doesn't stop her purchasing look-alike items too. "I enjoy collecting vintage bottles of Chanel No. 5, which we know Marilyn used to enjoy wearing. I also like items that are similar to those she owned in her household, of which the most recent item I purchased was a vintage Mexican tile, the same as those Marilyn had in her kitchen."

One of the biggest collectors of Marilyn's personal belongings is Scott Fortner. Like many other Marilyn Monroe fans, Scott began by collecting anything related to the star: "Incredibly, I still have the first piece of memorabilia I ever bought, which was a wall poster with many photos of Marilyn in a huge collage. I bought it at a souvenir store at Knott's Berry Farm in Los Angeles, when I was about thirteen years old. I started collecting Marilyn Monroe–owned items in 2001. Of course, I'd followed all of the news surrounding the sale of Marilyn's estate items at Christie's in 1999, but the closest I could get to that auction was the issue of *People* magazine with the cover story all about it.

"Not long after the Christie's auction, I started to notice Marilyn Monroe estate items coming up for sale on eBay,

OPPOSITE: When Marilyn appears on a magazine cover, fans flock to pick up a copy.

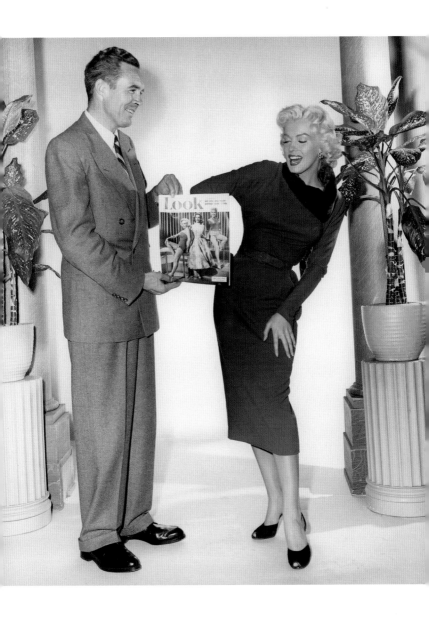

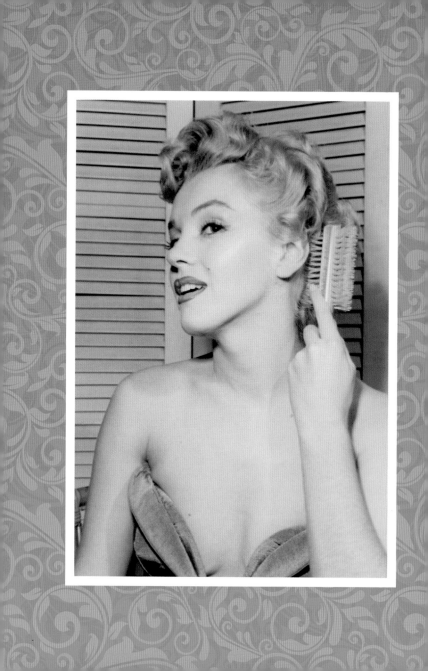

and I started buying. The first Marilyn-owned item I purchased was her personal script for a play titled *Maiden Voyage* by Paul Osborne. Theatrical producer Kermit Bloomgarden invited Marilyn to appear in the lead role of Athena on Broadway. She ultimately turned down the opportunity, but the script does have several annotations in her hand, and she wrote her initials on the first page. It was quite exciting to own an item from Marilyn's estate, and that's what started it all."

LIFE THROUGH OBJECTS

Marilyn's life can be seen in many ways, but perhaps the most intriguing is through the lens of her personal belongings. These five items shine a little light on the real woman behind the Hollywood icon.

1. CANDID PHOTOGRAPH

This photo is of Marilyn in 1946, when she was twenty years old. It shows the starlet in an outfit of white long-sleeved shirt, pencil skirt, and thick belt. Marilyn had just signed her first deal with Twentieth Century Fox, was full of hope for the future, and had her brunette hair dyed blonde. If

OPPOSITE: Even locks of Marilyn's hair have been sold at auction.

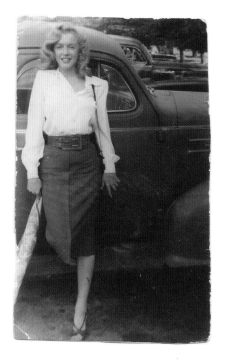

ever there was a photograph that shows just how much Marilyn was looking forward to the future, this is it. The actress kept this picture in her personal collection while living at the home of her foster mother, Ana Lower. She later gave it and several others to her boyfriend, Bill Pursel. Pursel was a university student and stuck the photograph to his cork board. The pinhole can still be seen just above the car roof, to the right of Marilyn's head.

2. BOOKSHOP RECEIPT

Marilyn was an avid reader and frequented the Beverly Hills branch of Martindale's bookstore regularly. Rachel Brand, the manager of Martindale's, told journalists in 1954 that she was a serious customer. "Marilyn is a great reader. Marilyn has been a great reader since way back, long before she was Marilyn Monroe. She reads Kafka, Thomas Mann, and authors like that—no cheap stuff."

This receipt, dated October 29, 1958, was for two books: *Dance to the Piper* by Agnes De Mille and *The Great Gatsby* by F. Scott Fitzgerald. These were bought while Marilyn was making *Some Like it Hot* with Jack Lemmon and Tony Curtis. The film was not an easy one to make. Marilyn often suffered from stage fright and kept cast and crew waiting as a result. She was also pregnant, though sadly she miscarried shortly after the film was completed. However, while shooting was fraught with difficulties, the finished work is a masterpiece and is considered one of Marilyn's best films. The American Film Institute named it the greatest comedy of all time in 2000, and in a poll among hundreds of film critics conducted by the BBC in 2017, the movie's ranking among cinematic laugh-fests was upheld.

3. SHOT GLASS

Marilyn often became friends with crew members she met while on the set of her films. One of these was Twentieth Century Fox electrician James A. Gough. Gough knew Marilyn for many years, and when she moved into her Fifth Helena Drive home, the actress asked if he could stop by and check her wiring. He traveled to Brentwood one Saturday morning with his son Jim, who remembered that Marilyn

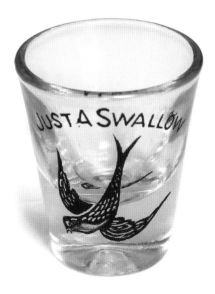

was in a happy mood, working in the garden. The small group had lunch together, and Marilyn showed off her new discovery: the Mexican tiles found beneath a layer of plaster in her living room. During a tour of the home, James noticed Marilyn's small collection of shot glasses and told her that he enjoyed buying those, too. In response, she picked up two identical glasses, bearing the words "Just a Swallow" and a picture of the bird. James was asked which of the two he would like, and then Marilyn handed him one and returned the other to her cabinet. James treasured the glass for the rest of his life.

189

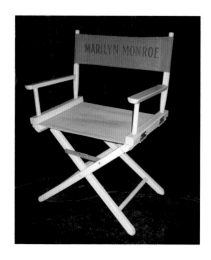

4. DIRECTOR'S CHAIR

Many actors and actresses had to sit on boxes and props while working on a film set, and some pictures of Marilyn show that this was the case for her, too. However, there is photographic evidence that by 1954, Marilyn had her own director's chair on the sets of *There's No Business Like Show Business* and *The Seven Year Itch*. This was considered a privilege, especially since director's chairs came complete with the actor's name printed on the back and nobody else was expected to sit there. This chair was given to Marilyn on the

OPPOSITE: Marilyn poses for a publicity photo while sitting in her director's chair.

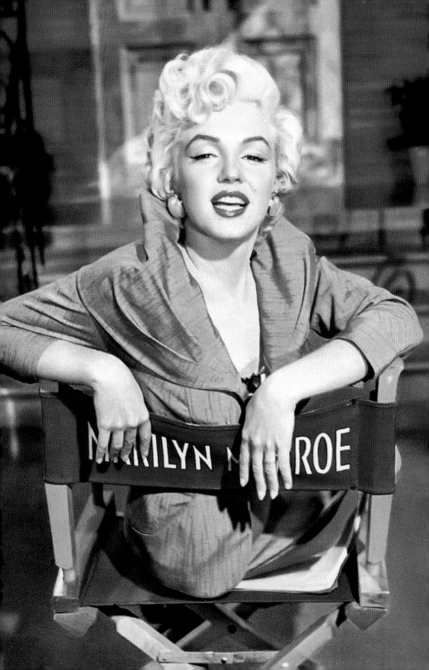

set of *Bus Stop* in 1956. It now resides in the collection of fan club president Greg Schreiner and is the only Marilyn Monroe director's chair known to still exist.

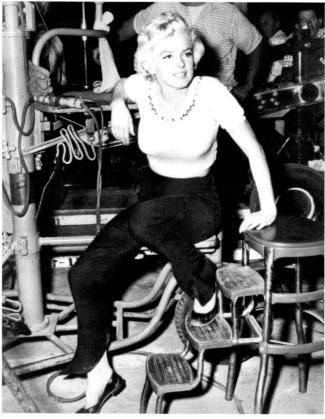

When she wasn't sitting in her own chair, Marilyn could be seen perched on steps and pieces of camera equipment.

5. MARILYN MONROE PRODUCTIONS MATCHBOOK

Marilyn's biggest wish was to be taken seriously as an actress and have the freedom to work on projects that she actually wanted to do. During the 1950s, the idea of a woman taking charge of her career was laughed at, particularly when that woman was known as a glamorous blonde with a sex-pot image. Marilyn did not want to be typecast or play in musicals for her entire career, so in 1954, after the breakdown of her marriage to Joe DiMaggio, she left Hollywood in search of a better life in New York.

Manhattan promised many wonderful experiences, including the opportunity to attend plays and act in theater. It also offered her creative independence with the formation of her own film company, Marilyn Monroe Productions. Marilyn and photographer Milton Greene were the major shareholders, and together they planned to "make good pictures." The 1957 movie *The Prince and the Showgirl* was made under

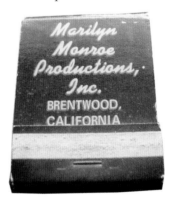

the MMP umbrella, before the two went their separate ways shortly thereafter. This matchbook was designed for the company, and it is interesting to note that while MMP was formed in New York, the matchbook's address is Marilyn's last residence of Brentwood, since she still owned the company at the time of her death.

MEXICAN TILES

Marilyn's love of Mexican home furnishings was abundantly evident in the bright, colorful, and distinctive tiles displayed all over her Fifth Helena Drive home. The house also boasted four Latin-inscribed tiles outside the front door, bearing the words *Cursum Perficio*. Translated this means "I finish my journey." These and the Mexican tiles remain a continuing source of inspiration for Marilyn's admirers.

Longtime devotee Hanna Nixon is so fascinated by the tiles that she makes replicas for herself and others. "Each tile is made to order for the customer," Hanna says. "They know each one has been lovingly made just for them." Hanna currently makes replicas of the interior tiles, as well as two versions of the *Cursum Perficio* tiles. "Nothing says Marilyn to me more than the items she personally

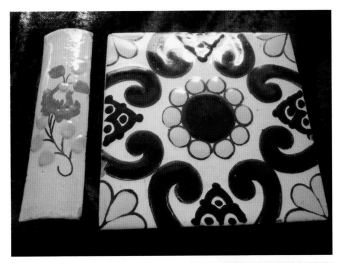

FROM TOP: Original tiles from
Marilyn's last home. • A replica
tile created by Marilyn fan
Hanna Nixon.

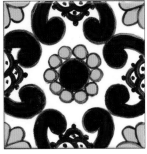

chose on her trip to Mexico for
her little hacienda home, with
bright colors and bold patterns.
Just looking at the tiles now, in
use in my own home, I am reminded of her."

Hanna's tiles are available from her Facebook page,
Marilyn's Mexican Home. Here Hanna shows us how to
produce the flower tile, which was displayed above Marilyn's bathtub.

MAKE YOUR OWN MEXICAN TILE

WHAT YOU'LL NEED

- ○ **One plain, glazed tile**
- ○ **Pencil**
- ○ **Ceramic paints**
- ○ **Tissues**
- ○ **Kiln or oven**

1) Using photographs of the image you wish to create, draw a template the same size as your tile. You may want to practice with different designs and colors to perfect your technique.

2) Take a plain, glazed tile and make sure it is clean and free of dust. Use your template to carefully draw the elements of the flower onto the tile with a

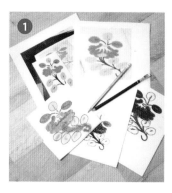
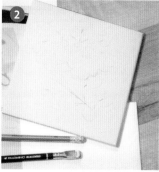

pencil. Make sure you leave enough room around it so that the paint (in step 3) does not spill over the sides of the tile.

3) Using ceramic paints, carefully fill the design with a small paintbrush. You will need brown/black paint for the stems and yellow and deep orange for the petals. Gently erase any visible pencil marks with a tissue and allow the tile to dry for twenty-four hours.

4) Bake in a kiln or oven according to the paint manufacturer's instructions, and let the tile cool in the oven overnight.

5) Your completed tile is now ready for display!

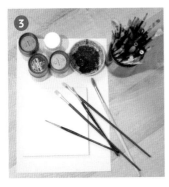

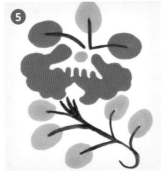

SEVEN

walk with Marilyn

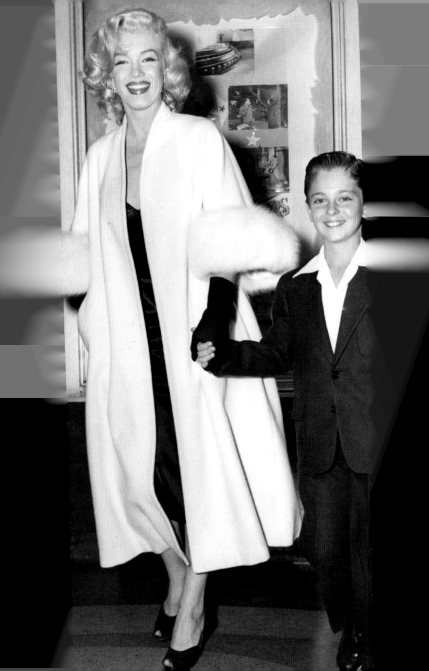

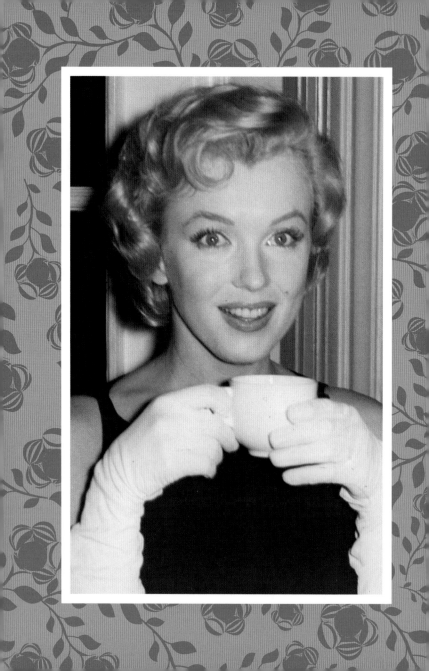

ALTHOUGH MARILYN WAS A DOWN-TO-EARTH woman, she did still enjoy the finer things in life, such as shopping in fancy stores and eating in beautiful restaurants. Shopping without a disguise could often be problematic, and photos taken by photographer Sam Shaw show Marilyn perusing items in a department store while crowds of fans stare in through the window. Indeed, while she was shopping in London in 1956, the public's fascination became so intense that the police had to be called to clear the road. It is easy to see why Marilyn often wore a dark wig and an old coat in hopes of gaining some degree of privacy.

Dining out was less stressful because fans were kept out of most restaurants and bars, but that did not stop them from surrounding Marilyn once she left. And there were still occasions when the actress was stared at by other diners inside the building. It also wasn't unusual for waiters to come up and request autographs between courses.

While many of Marilyn's haunts no longer exist, there are still some restaurants and shopping locations that remain thriving. Here are some of the locations you can visit.

OPPOSITE: Fans still flock to restaurants where Marilyn ate and drank. Here she is seen drinking tea while in London. PREVIOUS SPREAD: Marilyn out on the town with *River of No Return* costar Tommy Rettig.

THE POLO LOUNGE

**The Beverly Hills Hotel, 9641 Sunset Boulevard,
Beverly Hills, CA 90210**

Located in the famous Beverly Hills Hotel, the Polo Lounge was the place to see and be seen and is still regularly host to the rich and famous. Marilyn stayed at the hotel frequently, including during the 1960 filming of *Let's Make Love*, so it was inevitable that the Polo Lounge would become a favorite haunt. Sporting a candy-striped ceiling and a separate patio area, the restaurant remains reminiscent of the golden days of Hollywood, with intimate booths and alcoves as well as convenient tables from which to people-watch.

BARNEY'S BEANERY

8447 Santa Monica Boulevard, West Hollywood, CA 90069

Established in 1920, the original Barney's Beanery is a sight to behold. With vintage memorabilia decorating the walls and booths, this funky restaurant is incredibly popular with Marilyn fans. The woman herself often ate at Barney's when she was a student at the Actors Lab, and it is also believed that she came here after posing for her famous nude calendar photographs in 1949. The place is full of history. To give a perspective on how old it actually is: Marilyn's idol, Jean Harlow, was a frequent guest in the 1930s.

THE MUSSO & FRANK GRILL

6667 Hollywood Boulevard, Hollywood, CA 90028

This restaurant opened in 1919 and is still going strong. Dripping glamour and sophistication, the Musso & Frank

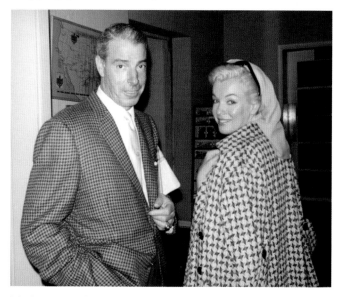

Marilyn and Joe DiMaggio out on a date.

Grill played host to Marilyn throughout her career. Notable visits were during her starlet days, when she dined with fellow acting students, and during her courtship and marriage to Joe DiMaggio, when they could eat quietly without the intrusion of fans. Food served during this time would have included minced chicken with noodles au gratin and corned beef and cabbage.

After you've finished eating, you can pop across the road to Larry Edmunds Bookshop, which has been in business for over seventy years. It is not known whether the store played host to Marilyn, but it is filled with some fabulously rare books about her, so it is well worth a visit.

THE RAINBOW BAR AND GRILL

9015 Sunset Boulevard, West Hollywood, CA 90069

When Marilyn agreed to meet DiMaggio on a blind date, it took place at the Villa Nova restaurant, which has since become the Rainbow Bar and Grill. On the date, Marilyn wore a blue suit with white silk blouse and ate a bowl of spaghetti. Popular with Monroe fans, the restaurant still serves pasta (and much more) and boasts wood-paneled walls and red-leather booths. Legend has it that Marilyn and Joe dined at table 14. Other famous customers included Judy Garland, Charlie Chaplin, and Dean Martin.

SARDI'S

234 West Forty-Fourth Street, New York, NY 10036

One of New York's most famous restaurants, this legendary location has been greeting diners for ninety years. Marilyn ate at Sardi's frequently during the mid-1950s and was even photographed inside the restaurant during a break from location filming for *The Seven Year Itch* and while celebrating the birthday of actress Susan Strasberg. Sardi's is famous for the caricatures of actors and actresses displayed on its walls and even has a gift shop where tourists can purchase related memorabilia.

21 CLUB

21 West Fifty-Second Street, New York, NY 10019

First opened during the Prohibition era, the 21 Club is a former speakeasy that is now known as a hangout for actors, sports stars, and of course Marilyn. Hanging from the ceiling in the famous 21 Bar Room are gifts from many famous stars, and the walls are lined with photographs and memorabilia representative of times gone by.

Marilyn attended a party here while in New York for *The Seven Year Itch* and was a frequent patron after moving to the Big Apple in late 1954. It was at 21 that Marilyn first met photographer Eve Arnold, who would go on to photograph the actress many times, including while shooting *The Misfits* in 1960.

FARMERS MARKET

6333 West Third Street, Los Angeles, CA 90036

Opened in 1934, this historic food market has been popular with celebrities for over eighty years. The last birthday cake Marilyn ever received—on the set of *Something's Got to Give* in June 1962—was purchased from the Farmers Market, but perhaps her most famous association came eleven years earlier, in 1951. Voted Miss Cheesecake by *Stars and Stripes* magazine, Marilyn traveled to the Farmers Market and visited Michael's Cheesecake stall, where she wore a bathing costume, lacy apron, and chef's hat. Photos of

OPPOSITE: Wherever she went, Marilyn had the ability to light up a room.

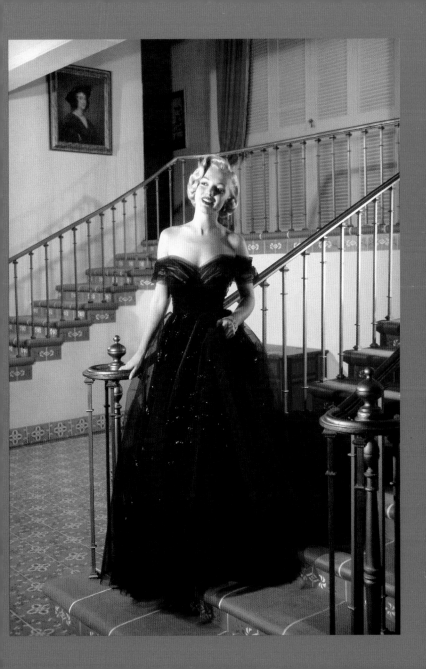

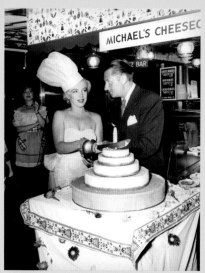

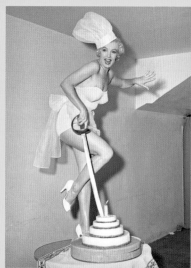

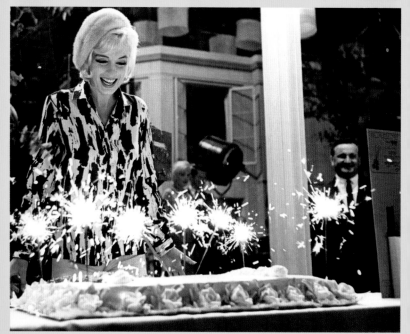

the event show Marilyn balanced on a table, slicing into a giant cheesecake with a sword, and then tasting it from her finger.

OLVERA STREET

Los Angeles, CA 90012

The most famous historic street in Los Angeles, Olvera, is a colorful array of Mexican stalls selling everything from musical instruments and puppets to clothing and housewares. It is likely that Marilyn visited this location many times during her life, but one specific visit happened in December 1961—Marilyn's last Christmas—when she bought tree decorations with Joe DiMaggio. The street would have also been of great interest to Marilyn when she bought her Fifth Helena Drive home, since she could easily buy Mexican knickknacks from here. Olvera Street is located just across the road from Union Station, where Marilyn traveled to and from Los Angeles on numerous occasions.

OPPOSITE, TOP: Marilyn makes a publicity appearance at the Farmers Market. BOTTOM: The last birthday cake Marilyn ever received was from the Farmers Market.

SAKS FIFTH AVENUE

9600 Wilshire Boulevard, Beverly Hills, CA 90212
611 Fifth Avenue, New York, NY 10022

Marilyn shopped in the Beverly Hills Saks Fifth Avenue store regularly, and in the early days of her career, agent Johnny Hyde would bring her there in order to buy clothes. On leaving California for the East Coast, the actress transferred her affections to the New York branch, where she was seen frequently during her marriage to Arthur Miller.

BLOOMINGDALE'S

1000 Third Avenue, Fifty-Ninth Street and Lexington Avenue, New York, NY 10022

Another department store adored by Marilyn was Bloomingdale's and, in particular, its flagship store at Fifty-Ninth Street in New York City. She once came here with actress Susan Strasberg and, according to Susan, was wearing no underclothes when she tried on new outfits. Marilyn would have no doubt been intrigued to learn that in 1983, Bloomingdale's showcased a Remembering Marilyn collection of capri pants and dresses, all inspired by the actress.

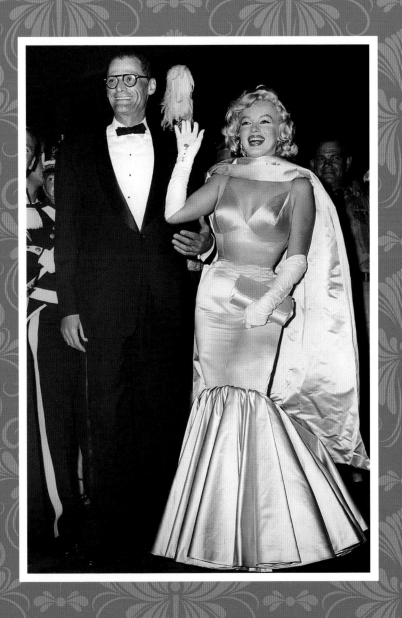

resources

FASHION/BEAUTY

Allyson Scanlon: iconicdresses.co.uk and
    iconicdresses.patternbyetsy.com

Anello & Davide: handmadeshoes.co.uk

Bettylicious: bettylicious.co.uk

Boots: boots.com

Chanel: chanel.com

Charlotte Tilbury: charlottetilbury.com

Collectif: collectif.co.uk

Cornelia James: corneliajames.com

Dawn Gray (Marilyn bag and hat decoration designer):
    @mmwritergirl (Twitter and Instagram)

Elizabeth Arden: elizabetharden.co.uk

Emilio Pucci: emiliopucci.com

Emmpress Sparkle (crocheted dolls):
    @emmpress_sparkle (Instagram)

Erno Laszlo: ernolaszlo.com

Esther Smith: morningstarpinup.com,
    @morningstar_pinup (Instagram)

Esther Williams: esther-williams.com

Ferragamo: ferragamo.com

Floris: florislondon.com

Gap: gap.com

Glamour Bunny: glamourbunny.com

Hanna Nixon Mexican Tiles: Marilyn's Mexican Home on Facebook
    (facebook.com/groups/675821142560639)

Lindy Bop: lindybop.co.uk

M.A.C.: maccosmetics.com

Max Factor: maxfactor.com

Pinup Girl Clothing: pinupgirlclothing.com

Revlon: revlon.com

Sexy Hair: sexyhair.com

Soap and Glory: soapandglory.com

Stop Staring!: stopstaringclothing.com

Victoria's Secret: victoriassecret.com

What Katie Did: whatkatiedid.com

TRIBUTE ARTISTS

Ashley Clark: castingashley.com, @ashleyasmarilyn (Instagram)

Blonde Fox Entertainment: @emilygorgeous13 (Instagram)

Hanna Nixon: unmistakablymarilyn.co.uk

Jessica "Sugar" Kiper: @sugarkiper and @americon.monroe
    (Instagram)

Kaity Kinloch: marilynperforms.com, @marilynperforms (Instagram)

Kaylie Minzola: @marilynminzola (Instagram)

Mariam Myrone: @mariammyrone and @marilyn.m_style
    (Instagram)

Suzie Kennedy: suziekennedy.com, @suziekennedy (Instagram)

MARILYN MONROE WEBSITES

The Marilyn Monroe Collection: themarilynmonroecollection.com, @
    marilynmonroecollection (Instagram)

Marilyn Remembered: marilynremembered.com,
    @marilynremembered (Instagram)

credits

Courtesy Photofest: Pages 16 (left), 16 (right), 17, 22, 43, 53, 55, 71 (left), 74 (left), 74 (right), 77, 83 (left), 113 (left) 113 (middle), 113 (right), 114 (left), 115 (left), 115 (right), 126, 159, 164, 169, 171, 174, 181 (right), 199, 207, 215

Courtesy Everett Collection, Inc.: Pages 13, 23, 25 (bottom), 26, 36, 41 (left), 41 (right), 61, 69 (left), 76, 80, 83 (bottom right), 88, 90, 117, 128, 131, 150, 161, 180, 184, 192, 200, 203, 208 (left)

Courtesy author's collection: Page 186

Courtesy Kim Goodwin: Page 18

All other Marilyn Monroe photos courtesy the **David Wills Collection**

Greg Schreiner photos by Jay Jorgensen

Jessica "Sugar" Kiper photos by Glenn Campbell, GlennCampbellPhoto.com; makeup by Adam Christopher

Kaity Kinloch portrait by Deb McDonald

Laura Kallio (wearing designs by Esther Smith) photos by Brian Kallio

Makeup and hair tutorials photos by Bernard Hales, tutorials by Suzie Kennedy

Mariam Myrone photos by Oleg Mironov

Marisa Vanderpest photos by Jim Parson

Purse and hat decoration tutorials photos by Michael Finn, designs by Dawn Gray

Tile tutorial photos by Martin Nickless, tutorial by Hanna Nixon

Vanessa Roden photo by Chloe Roden

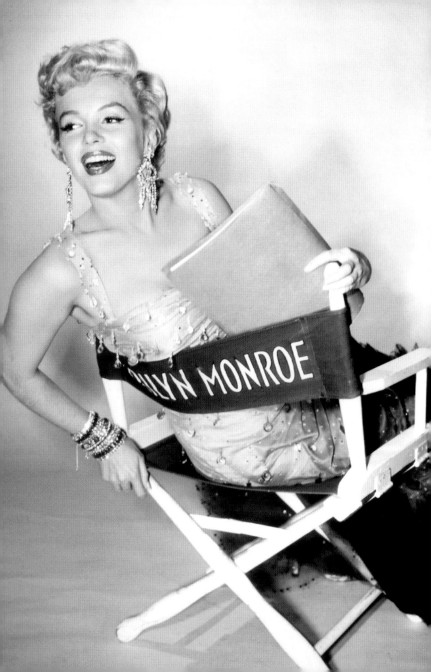

acknowledgments

I would like to thank everyone who shared thoughts and photographs for this book. Suzie Kennedy, Dawn Gray, and Hanna Nixon created terrific tutorials. Thanks especially to Aunty Dawn for creating the flower tutorial on such short notice and to my dad for taking the pictures. Bernard Hales took some of the best photos of Suzie Kennedy that I have ever seen, and I am immensely grateful to him as well as to Joan for opening their home to us and being so gracious. Thanks also to Bernard for countless other photo favors. David Wills graciously opened up his photo archives to me, and I am eternally grateful.

To my agent, Piers Blofeld, and my editor, Cindy Sipala: I am so happy to work with you both and can't wait for our future projects.

To my family, Mum, Dad, Paul, Wendy, and Angelina, and my friends Claire and Helen: I am always so grateful for your support and unconditional love.

My husband, Richard, and daughter, Daisy, have always been an inspiration to me. Their love knows no bounds, and for that I am immensely grateful.

And finally, my thanks must go to Marilyn and everyone who still admires her. Without Marilyn and the love she continues to provoke in people, this book would have no meaning.